Dedicated to

All those women who suffer in silence with urinary incontinence and equally to the concerned enthusiastic healthcare professionals who find a complete solution to the best effect relieving patients

Understandi[ng] Female Urinary Inc[ontinence] and Master Management

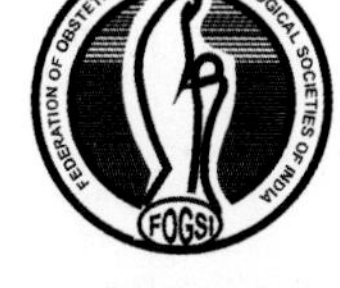

Federation of Obstetric and Gynaecological Societies of India

Understanding
Female Urinary Incontinence
and Master Management

Editor

Prakash Trivedi

MD DGO FCPS DNB FICMCH Dip. in Pelviscopic Surgery (Germany)
Dip. in Hysteroscopic Surgery (France) Fellowship in ART (Australia and Singapore)
Fellowship in Urogynaecology (Australia and USA)
Professor and Head
Department of Obstetrics and Gynecology, Rajawadi Municipal Hospital
Scientific Director
National Institute of Laser and Endoscopic Surgery (NILES) and
Aakar IVF-ICSI Centre, Saakar Urinary Incontinence Centre
Dr Trivedi's Total Health Care Centre
Gynecologic Endoscopist, Urogynecologist and ART Consultant
Jaslok Hospital and Bhabha Atomic Research Centre Hospital
Mumbai, Maharashtra, India
President (2013-2015)
Indian Association of Gynaecological Endoscopists

Co-editor

Ajay Rane

MBBS MSc MD FRCS FRCOG FRANZCOG CU FICOG (Hon) PhD
Professor and Head
Department of Obstetrics and Gynecology
Consultant and Urogynecologist
James Cook University, Townsville, Queensland, Australia
Vice President
The Royal Australian and New Zealand College of Obstetricians and
Gynaecologists (RANZCOG)

Forewords

Shirish S Sheth, CN Purandare

A FOGSI Publication

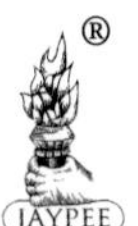

JAYPEE BROTHERS MEDICAL PUBLISHERS (P) LTD

New Delhi • London • Philadelphia • Panama

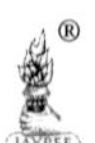

Jaypee Brothers Medical Publishers (P) Ltd.

Headquarters

Jaypee Brothers Medical Publishers (P) Ltd.
4838/24, Ansari Road, Daryaganj
New Delhi 110 002, India
Phone: +91-11-43574357
Fax: +91-11-43574314
Email: jaypee@jaypeebrothers.com

Overseas Offices

J.P. Medical Ltd.
83, Victoria Street, London
SW1H 0HW (UK)
Phone: +44-2031708910
Fax: +02-03-0086180
Email: info@jpmedpub.com

Jaypee-Highlights Medical Publishers Inc.
City of Knowledge, Bld. 237, Clayton
Panama City, Panama
Phone: +507-301-0496
Fax: +507-301-0499
Email: cservice@jphmedical.com

Jaypee Medical Inc.
The Bourse
111, South Independence Mall East
Suite 835, Philadelphia, PA 19106, USA
Phone: + 267-519-9789
Email: joe.rusko@jaypeebrothers.com

Jaypee Brothers Medical Publishers (P) Ltd.
17/1-B, Babar Road, Block-B
Shaymali, Mohammadpur
Dhaka-1207, Bangladesh
Mobile: +08801912003485
Email: jaypeedhaka@gmail.com

Jaypee Brothers Medical Publishers (P) Ltd.
Shorakhute
Kathmandu, Nepal
Phone: +00977-9841528578
Email: jaypee.nepal@gmail.com

Website: www.jaypeebrothers.com
Website: www.jaypeedigital.com

Inquiries for bulk sales may be solicited at: jaypee@jaypeebrothers.com

Understanding Female Urinary Incontinence and Master Management

First Edition: **2014**

ISBN : 978-93-5090-734-4

Printed at: S. Narayan & Sons

Contributors

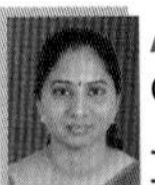
A Tamilselvi
Clinical Fellow
James Cook University
Townsville, Queensland, Australia

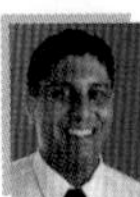
Ajay Rane MBBS MSc MD FRCS FRCOG FRANZCOG CU FICOG (Hon) PhD
Professor and Head
Department of Obstetrics and Gynecology
Consultant Urogynecologist
James Cook University
Townsville, Queensland, Australia
Vice President
The Royal Australian and New Zealand College of Obstetricians and Gynaecologists (RANZCOG)

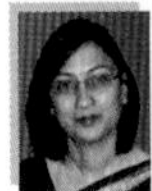
Amita Jain MS (Obs and Gynae)
Fellowship in Urogynaecology (Australia)
Consultant Urogynecologist
Division of Urogynecology
Medanta Kidney and Urology Institute
Medanta Vattikuti Institute of Robotic Surgery
Gurgaon, Haryana, India

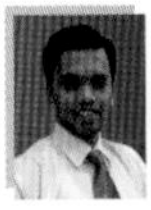
Animesh Gandhi MS DGO DNB (Obs and Gynae)
Junior Clinical Associate
Dr Trivedi's Total Health Care Centre
Mumbai, Maharashtra, India

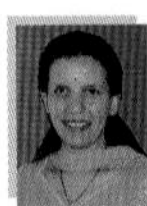
Anita Patel MS MCh DNB FRCS
Urogynecologist
Endoskopik Klinik and Hospital
Shivaji Park, Mahim (W)
Mumbai, Maharashtra, India
Muljibhai Patel Hospital
Nadiad, Gujarat, India

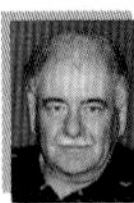
Ian P Tucker MBBS (Adel) FRCOG FRANZCOG
Urogynecologist
Vice President
Continence Foundation of Australia
Member
Advisory Board
Urogynaecological Society of Australasia

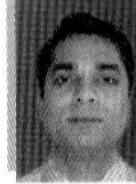
Jay Iyer MD DNB MRCOG FRANZCOG
Senior Lecturer
Department of Obstetrics and Gynecology
James Cook University
Townsville, Queensland, Australia

Li-Tsa Koh
Urology Fellow
Department of Urology
Concord Repatriation General Hospital
Department of Urology
Concord Hospital Clinical School
Sydney, Australia

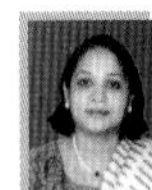
Madhuri Gandhi DGO DNB (Obs and Gynae)
Department of Obstetrics and Gynecology
AL Ahli Hospital
Doha, Qatar
Junior Clinical Associate
Dr Trivedi's Total Health Care Centre
Mumbai, Maharashtra, India

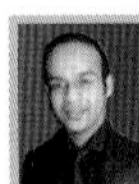
Mohit Saraogi MBBS MS
Registrar
Seth Gordhandas Sunderdas Medical College
King Edward Memorial Hospital
Mumbai, Maharashtra, India

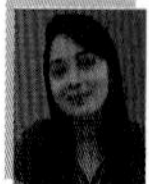
Nishita Parekh DNB
(Obs and Gynae)
Junior Clinical Associate
Dr Trivedi's Total Health Care Centre
Mumbai, Maharashtra, India

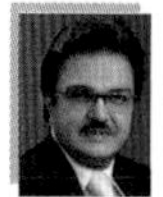
Prakash Trivedi MD DGO FCPS DNB
Professor and Head
Department of Obstetrics and Gynecology, Rajawadi Hospital
Scientific Director
National Institute of Laser and Endoscopic Surgery(NILES) and Aakar IVF-ICSI Centre, Saakar Urinary Incontinence Centre,
Dr Trivedi's Total Health Care Centre
Gynaec Endoscopist
Jaslok Hospital and Bhabha Atomic Research Centre Hospital
Mumbai, Maharashtra, India
President (2013-2015)
Indian Association of Gynaecological Endoscopists

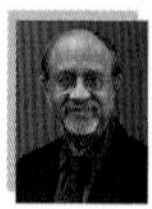
RM Saraogi MD FICOG FCPS DGO
Honorary and Head
Department of Obstetrics and Gynecology
RN Cooper Hospital
Honorary Professsor
Seth Gordhandas Sunderdas Medical College and King Edward Memorial Hospital
Mumbai, Maharashtra, India

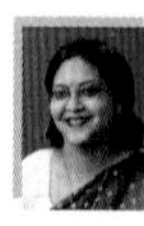
Rooma Sinha MD DNB MNAMS
Consultant Gynecologist
Laparoscopic and Robotic Surgeon and Urogynecologist
Apollo Hospital
Hyderabad, Andhra Pradesh, India

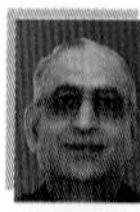
S Mahadevan MD DGO FRCOG
Gynecologist
Pembury Hospital
Kent, UK

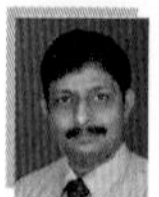
Sandeep Patil DNB MNAMS
(Obs and Gynae)
Senior Clinical Associate
Dr Trivedi's Total Health Care Centre
Mumbai, Maharashtra, India

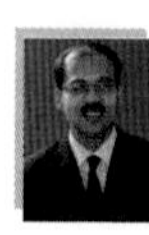
Sanjay Sinha MS MCh MAMS
Consultant Urologist and Transplant Surgeon
Apollo Hospital
Hyderabad, Andhra Pradesh, India
Chair
IUGA Exchange Steering Committee (IESC)

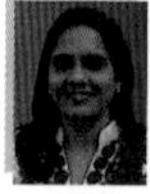
Sarika Dodwani MD DNB
(Obs and Gynae)
Junior Clinical Associate
Dr Trivedi's Total Health Care Centre
Mumbai, Maharashtra, India

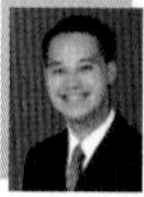
Vincent Tse MBBS MS (Syd) FRACS (Urol)
Consultant Urologist
Concord Repatriation General Hospital, Sydney, Australia
Clinical Senior Lecturer
Concord Hospital Clinical School
University of Sydney, Australia

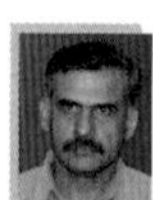
Vivek Joshi MD
Consultant Gynecologist
King Edward Memorial Hospital
Pune, Maharashtra, India

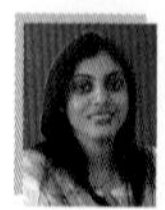
Yugali Warade DNB
(Obs and Gynae)
Junior Clinical Associate
Dr Trivedi's Total Health Care Centre
Mumbai, Maharashtra, India

Dr. Shirish S. Sheth

M.D., F.R.C.O.G. (Ad Eundem), F.A.C.O.G. (Hon.), F.A.C.S., F.I.C.S., F.C.P.S., F.I.C.O.G., F.A.M.S., F.S.O.G.C.

Consultant Gynaecologist

Breach Candy Hospital • Sir Hurkisondas Hospital • Saifee Hospital

Foreword

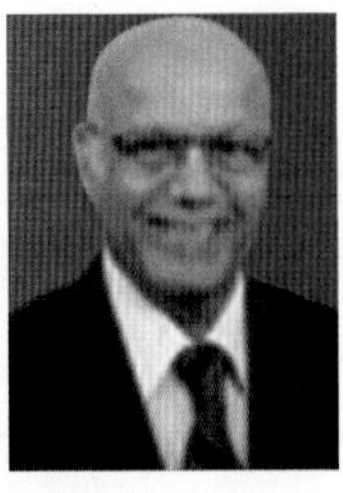

It is indeed an honor for me to write the foreword and a matter of pride for FOGSI to publish much-needed literature on 'understanding' of the ill-understood subject of urinary incontinence and 'mastering' its management.

The book distinctly defines the anatomical and neuroanatomical aspects, and the role that urodynamics and imaging play in understanding the complexities. Dr Anita Patel, Dr RM Saraogi and others have amalgamated in lucid style, the multifactorial happenings of the subject, which will lead to productive reading to master the management.

Both the editors are deeply involved in the subject. Dr Prakash Trivedi, who is deeply involved with propagating knowledge on subject and Dr Ajay Rane from Australia, who leads the way for RANZCOG (The Royal Australian and New Zealand College of Obstetricians and Gynaecologists), have balanced their experience to elegantly cover this enigmatic dilemma and provide an authentic and comprehensive treatise on the subject. Despite the exciting surgical developments and confusing pathophysiology, the book helps in lending clarity on the topic to stimulate better management of urinary incontinence.

The book can be a beacon to all those colleagues treating and/or fumbling at the complaint of urinary dribble, its vagaries and orderly management. The book invites readers to make liberal use of scientific data with a rationale to choose and deliver well-balanced treatment.

Shirish S Sheth

MD FRCOG (Ad Eundem) FACOG (Hon)

FACS FICS FCPS FICOG FAMS FSOGC

Consultant Gynecologist

Breach Candy Hospital

Sir Hurkisondas Hospital

Saifee Hospital

Mumbai, Maharashtra, India

Former President FIGO (2000-2003)

Foreword

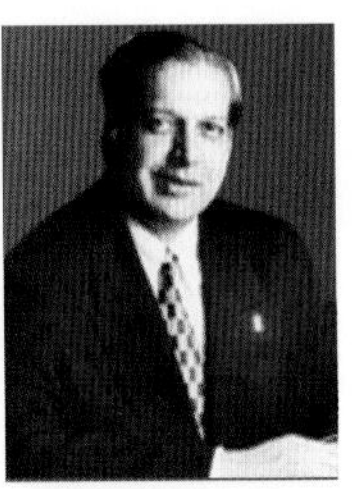

During my long career in Gynecology and Obstetrics of more than 3 decades, traveling in different parts of the world, I have come across authors and editors with high level of purpose.

Dr Prakash Trivedi, who has released around five to six books on Endoscopic Surgery, Assisted Reproductive Infertility Dilemma's Safe Minimal Access Surgery, etc. has a unique sense of passion, a clean directed message, involvement of other experts and most significant, the book is timed meticulous on the subject, which is needed by the medical community.

Apart from being a specialist and a good endoscopic surgeon, he has deep driving interest in pelvic floor and vaginal surgery. His special interest in Female Urinary Incontinence is of paramount interest not only to him, peers and colleagues but also for the patient.

The book *Understanding Female Urinary Incontinence and Master Management* [a Federation of Obstetric and Gynaecological Societies of India (FOGSI) Publication] covers almost all aspects needed on the subject from anatomy, physiology, neuroendocrinology, evaluations, medical and surgical treatments, and advances with innovations.

The co-editor Professor Ajay Rane, a Gynecologist well-established world authority in urogynecology from James Cook University, Australia, is a skilled surgeon as well as reputed teacher. He is a friend of FOGSI, many gynecologists and urologists all over the world. His contribution in the book is of immense scientific values for all readers and enthusiast in the subject.

I am sure that the knowledge and skills picked up from the book will help many women of all over the world. The book will be an asset for all FOGSI members.

CN Purandare
MD MA (Obs) DGO DFP D Obst RCPJ (Dub) FICOG
Hon Professor of Obstetrics and Gynecology
Grant Medical College and JJ Hospital
Mumbai, Maharashtra, India
President Elect FIGO
Past President FOGSI
Past President MOGS

Preface

Many health problems of the female are quiet often ignored by patients and doctors, and even consultants do not have complete knowledge to manage such problems. One such subject is female urinary incontinence, which remains elusive both for the gynecologists and urologists. Quite often, there is a myth that the other specialty must be managing more patients. The patient gets tossed from a general practitioner to a consultant or a quack or not attended at all.

A complete and comprehensive book was much needed to explain various types of urinary incontinence, their prevalence and methods to diagnose. A thorough knowledge of physiology, anatomy and neuroanatomy is needed, backed by good clinical evaluation and role of urodynamic video-cystometry.

The medical management, conventional, laparoscopic and sling surgeries, selections of right procedure, accurate operative steps, difficulties, complications, long-term outcomes, controversies about type of sling-tape or mesh. New restrictions, older options revived, sacral modulation, artificial urethral sphincter and bulking agents, all are covered in the book.

The team of contributors are experts in respective fields with unique arts of teaching, simplified with caution when needed.

Understanding Female Urinary Incontinence and Master Management—a FOGSI publication will go a long way to improve our care and approach towards female urinary incontinence.

We are indebted to Professor Shirish S Sheth and Dr CN Purandare, reputed teachers for their forewords.

Prakash Trivedi
Ajay Rane

Acknowledgments

The Editor and Co-editor are indebted to all the contributors for the book. We acknowledge the permission granted by the Federation of Obstetric and Gynaecological Societies of India (FOGSI) President office bearers to make the book as FOGSI Publication. The book would not have been possible without the meticulous hard work done by our clinical associates Dr Sandeep Patil, Dr Animesh Gandhi, Dr Yugali Warade, Dr Sarika Dodwani, Dr Madhuri Gandhi and Dr Nishita Parekh. The office secretaries Hemal Vasani and Sonali Nikam of Dr Trivedi's Total Health Care Centre, Mumbai, Maharashtra, India, and Mr K Ramesh (Mumbai Branch) of M/s Jaypee Brothers Medical Publishers (P) Ltd, New Delhi, India.

Finally, we would like to appreciate the faith, tolerance, support and sincere devotion, which Mrs Priti Trivedi and Dr Paula Rane have shown in all our endeavors including the book.

Contents

CHAPTER

1

Magnitude of Female Urinary Incontinence: A Health Problem

Prakash Trivedi

Introduction and Definitions

Urinary incontinence (UI), according to the International Continence Society[1] is defined as the involuntary loss of urine. It simultaneously exists as a symptom or complaint, sign, or finding and defined condition. Within the broad context of lower urinary tract symptoms (LUTS), UI is considered a storage symptom as opposed to a voiding symptom: "storage" refers to the filling phase of the micturition cycle, whereas "voiding" refers to the emptying phase.

The most commonly recognized subtypes of UI are stress urinary incontinence (SUI) (**Figures 1.1A to C**), urge urinary incontinence (UUI), and mixed urinary incontinence (MUI). SUI is the involuntary loss of urine associated with effort or physical exertion (e.g. sporting activities) or sneezing or coughing.

Urge urinary incontinence is the involuntary loss of urine associated with an involuntary detrusor contraction (**Figure 1.2**) and urgency, a sudden, compelling desire to pass urine that is difficult to defer.

Mixed urinary incontinence is a combination of the former two—the involuntary loss of urine associated with urgency and with effort or physical exertion or sneezing or coughing. Other types of UI include functional UI, related to inability to reach the toilet in an otherwise normal urinary system; overflow UI, resulting from bladder overdistention or retention; and enuresis, insensible and continuous incontinence. Symptoms and findings of UI often coexist with other, associated LUTS, including symptoms related to storage and voiding. Overactive bladder (OAB) syndrome is the constellation of multiple storage symptoms predicated by urinary urgency, usually accompanied by frequency and nocturia, with or without UUI, in the absence of urinary tract infection (UTI) or other obvious pathology. Frequency, urgency, and nocturia can also occur separately. Voiding symptoms

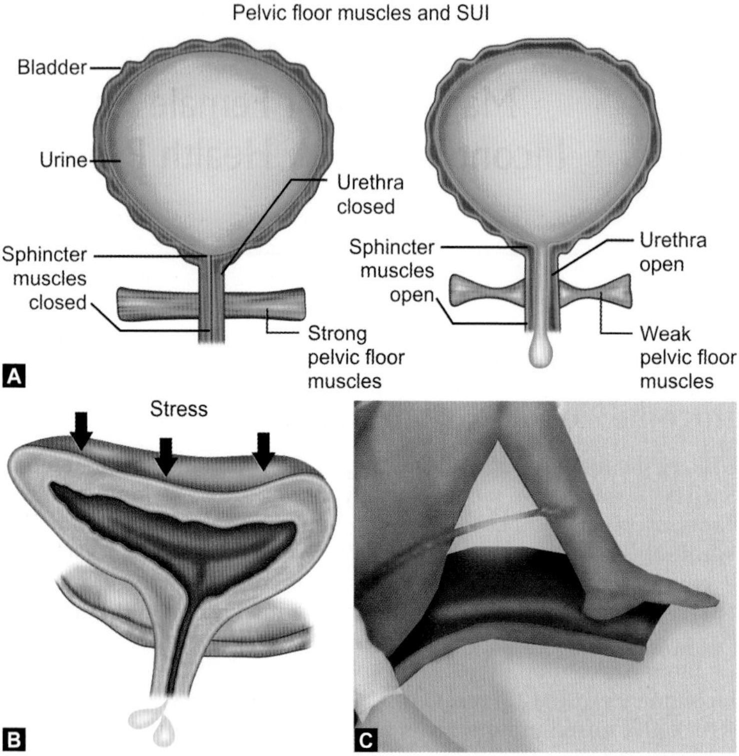

Pelvic floor muscles and SUI
Bladder
Urine
Urethra closed
Sphincter muscles closed
Strong pelvic floor muscles
Sphincter muscles open
Urethra open
Weak pelvic floor muscles
A
Stress
B
C

Figures 1.1A to C: Stress urinary incontinence

Large bladder muscle
Large bladder muscle contracting
Urine
Urine
Urethra, closed
Sphincter muscles, squeezed shut
Sphincter muscles, relaxed
Urethra, open

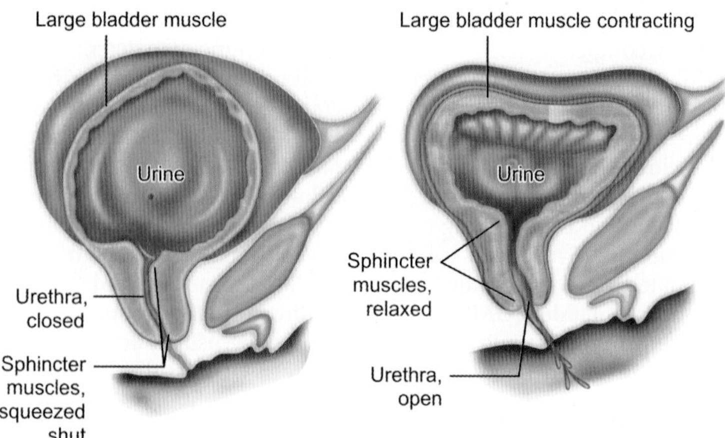

Figure 1.2: Involuntary detrusor contraction

that may coexist with UI include hesitancy, slow or weak urinary stream, straining to void, incomplete bladder emptying, dysuria, and retention. Pain, either specific to pelvic organs (e.g. bladder, urethra, vaginal, rectal/anal) or generalized, can also occur. Voiding dysfunction is a diagnosis made on the basis of symptoms and clinical findings and defined as abnormally slow or incomplete micturition, including acute or chronic urinary retention. It most typically occurs in women as an adverse outcome after invasive treatment for SUI or other pelvic floor conditions. UI and LUTS often occur in women in association with other pelvic floor conditions, including pelvic organ prolapse (POP). SUI is commonly found in women with POP, although as the degree of POP increases, SUI becomes less apparent, and other LUTS may develop. SUI can be demonstrated by reducing the POP and testing for SUI. When SUI is observed only after the reduction of coexistent prolapse, it is referred to as occult or potential SUI. Impact UI is a common condition in women. Estimates vary by definition, but approximately 25 to 75 percent of women report some UI.

In India, approximately 10 to 34 percent of surveyed women report some UI.[2,3] Extrapolation of prevalence based on prevalence studies in USA suggest that around 50 million Indian women suffer from UI.[4] Approximately 10 percent of women diagnosed with SUI undergo surgical correction.[5] SUI is the most common subtype of UI reported by women: about 57 percent of women with UI report SUI as the primary or sole symptom of incontinence. About 23 percent of women have UI and 20 percent have MUI.[2] Even when UI is recognized, a substantial number of women do not receive a formal diagnosis or do not seek treatment. As age increases, the risk of MUI and UUI increase, whereas the risk of SUI decreases. Although all subtypes of UI represent a significant burden to individuals and health care systems, SUI is the subtype that is most amenable to surgical treatment. The economic impact of UI and pelvic floor conditions is significant with huge expenditures on medications, surgical treatment and for routine care that includes protective pads and laundry services. Combined with lack of awareness about the condition spending continues to increase substantially for treatment of UI.

The pathophysiology underlying UI is often multifactorial and specific to the subtype of UI (i.e. SUI vs UUI). In UUI, detrusor overactivity or involuntary bladder contraction is the etiologic event that results in the incontinence episode. Causes for detrusor overactivity are varied and include:

- Neurologic injury (brain or spinal cord)
- Changes to lower urinary tract function
  - Aging
  - Hormone withdrawal

- Bladder outlet obstruction
- Idiopathic causes (most cases).

Neurologic injury typically results in the loss of voluntary control of voiding, which leads to an uncoordinated OAB (neurogenic bladder).

- For lesions of the cerebral cortex or basal ganglia (i.e. suprapontine) damage to the brain induces overactivity by reducing voluntary inhibition of voiding, while typically preserving sensation and coordination of the sphincter.
- For lesions below the brainstem, including the spinal cord, damage eliminates voluntary and coordinated control of voiding, resulting in detrusor overactivity mediated by spinal reflex pathways. Typically, loss of bladder sensation occurs, also coordination between detrusor contraction and urinary sphincter relaxation is lost (i.e. detrusor-sphincter dyssynergia).
- Neurologic damage to structures distal to the spinal cord, including nerve roots or peripheral nerves, also can result in bladder and lower urinary tract dysfunction. Crush injury to the pudendal nerve during labor and delivery is thought to contribute to SUI.
- Systemic conditions, such as multiple sclerosis, Diabetes mellitus, Tabes dorsalis, pernicious anemia, Guillain-Barré syndrome, poliomyelitis, multiple system atrophy can affect multiple components of the neurologic pathways, resulting in varied voiding abnormalities.
- In non-neurogenic situations, including idiopathic, detrusor overactivity can develop as a result of pathophysiologic changes to the bladder muscle, affecting contractility, and to the balance between motor and sensory innervation.

The effects of age, hormone withdrawal, bladder outlet obstruction, local hypoxia, or partial denervation on the bladder tend to promote detrusor contraction and overactivity. Hypersensitivity or oversensitivity of the afferent (i.e. sensory) nerves of the bladder may also trigger detrusor overactivity.

For SUI, different mechanisms contribute primarily to incontinence episodes:

- Changes to anatomic support—structural components
- Changes to function of the urethra and bladder neck.

Anatomical factors in part necessary for maintenance of urinary continence and prevention of urinary loss include:

- A healthy, functioning striated sphincter
- Well-vascularized urethral submucosal tissue
- Intact vaginal wall support.

When any of these factors are compromised, the urethra may not remain closed at rest or during increased abdominal pressure, and SUI ensues. Loss of vaginal or pelvic floor support to the urethra and bladder allows the urethra to "sag" inappropriately during periods of increased abdominal pressure (i.e. stress or strain): the proximal urethra rotates and descends away from its retropubic position. Urethral closure is prevented, and urinary leakage occurs. This change in urethral position is commonly described as hypermobility.

Primary urethral sphincter weakness independent of hypermobility (i.e. intrinsic sphincter deficiency) can also result in SUI. In this situation, coaptation of the urethral mucosa is lost, as a result of deficient sphincter mass or function or submucosal tissue cushions or both.

Traditionally, intrinsic sphincter deficiency and urethral hypermobility were viewed as dichotomous mechanisms for SUI; however, current understanding of the pathophysiology of SUI assigns these factors to a mechanistic continuum, whereby most women have a component of both factors.

Risk Factors

Multiple risk factors have been proposed and studied for the development of SUI in women. SUI is a multifactorial health condition with many contributing factors involved in the pathogenesis, risk factors that have been more widely studied. Among those listed, age, parity, vaginal delivery, forceps, surgery around bladder, cystocele repair with mesh, obesity, hormone replacement, diabetes, and family history have been reproducibly associated with increased risk of SUI across most studies.

References

1. Haylen BT, de Ridder D, Freeman RM, Swift SE, Berghmans B, Lee J, et al. An International Urogynecological Association (IUGA)/International Continence Society (ICS) joint report on the terminology for female pelvic floor dysfunction. Neurourol Urodyn. 2010;29(1):4-20.
2. Bodhare TN, Valsangkar S, Bele SD. An epidemiological study of urinary incontinence and its impact on quality of life among women aged 35 years and above in a rural area. Indian J Urol. 2010;26:353-8.
3. Singh Abha, Agrawal Priti, Sachdev Nanakram. Incidence and epidemiology of urinary incontinence in women. J Obstet Gynecol India. 2007;57(2):155-7.
4. http://www.rightdiagnosis.com/u/urinary_incontinence/stats-country.htm
5. Anger J, Weinberg A, Albo M, Smith AL, Kim JH, Rodriguez L, et al. Trends in surgical management of stress urinary incontinence among female Medicare beneficiaries. Urology. 2009;74:283-7.

CHAPTER

2

Anatomical Aspects of Urinary Incontinence: Clinical Applications

Sandeep Patil, Nishita Parekh, Prakash Trivedi

Urethral Anatomy (Figure 2.1)

The female urethra is approximately 4 cm, imbedded in the connective tissue supporting the anterior vagina.

The urethra is composed of an inner epithelial lining, a spongy submucosa, a middle smooth muscle layer, and outer fibroelastic connective tissue (**Figure 2.2**). The spongy submucosa contains rich vascular plexus that is responsible for providing adequate urethral occlusive pressure to create the washer effect, an important female

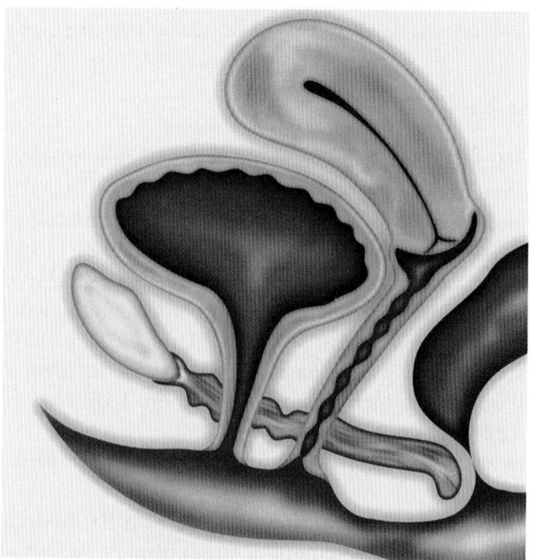

Figure 2.1: Normal micturition

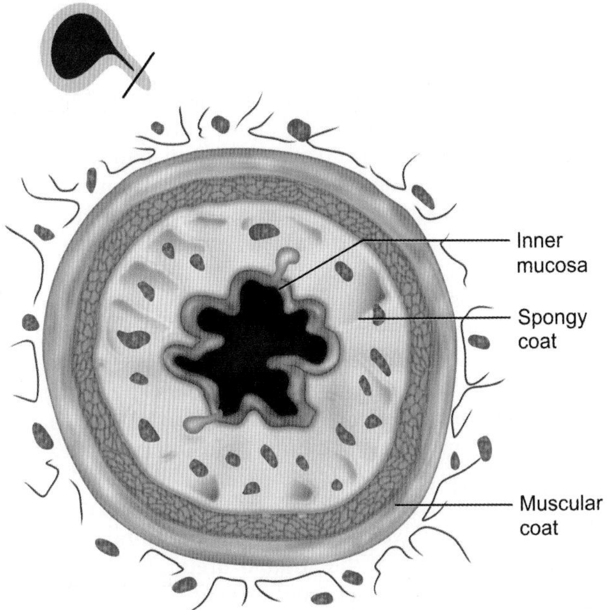

Figure 2.2: Cross-section of urethra

continence mechanism. Urethral smooth muscle and fibroelastic connective tissues circumferentially augment the occlusive pressure generated by the submucosa.

The female urethra is composed of four separate tissue layers that keep it closed. The inner mucosal lining keeps the urothelium moist and the urethra supple. The vascular spongy coat produces the mucus important in the mucosal seal mechanism. Compression from the middle muscular coat helps to maintain the resting urethral closure mechanism. The outer seromuscular layer augments the closure pressure provided by the muscular layer.

The urethral epithelium is composed of stratified squamous cells, which variably becomes transitional as the bladder is approached. The epithelium is arranged in longitudinal folds. At the base of the folds are scattered gland openings along the entire urethral length. The epithelium is supported by a loose lamina propria consisting of collagen fibrils and elastic fibers, arranged both circularly and longitudinally. A rich network of blood vessels is in the subepithelial layer.

The smooth muscle of the urethra is arranged longitudinally and obliquely with only a few circular fibers. The nerve supply is cholinergic and alpha-adrenergic. The longitudinal muscles may contribute to shortening and opening of the urethra during voiding. The oblique and circular fibers contribute to urethral closure at rest.

The striated urethral musculature is complex, and the components and their orientation are not agreed upon universally. The voluntary urethral sphincter really is a group of circular and loop-like inter-related muscle fibers, similar to that present in the anorectum. The innermost layer, which is prominent in the proximal two-thirds of the urethra, is the sphincter urethrae. More distally, the compressor urethrae and urethrovaginal sphincter are predominant.

These two muscles emanate from the anterolateral aspect of the distal half to one-third of the urethra and arch over the anterior or ventral surface. These striated muscles function as a unit. Because they are composed primarily of slow-twitch muscle fibers, these muscles serve ideally to maintain urethral tone. The muscles probably do maintain the urethral tone but contribute to voluntary closure and reflex closure of the urethra acutely during times of increased intra-abdominal pressure. The medial-most pubovisceral portion of the levator ani complex also is a major contributor to active bladder neck and urethral closure.

Histologic examination of the striated urethral sphincter indicates that for the most part, the muscle complex surrounds the urethra in an incomplete fashion. Fibers can be observed to be deficient along the posterior aspect of the urethra. The shape of the muscle complex can be described as resembling a horseshoe or an omega symbol.

Investigations using ultrasonographic imaging of the urethra also have confirmed a paucity of muscle bulk along the posterior urethra.[1] The urethral meatus empties into the vestibule after the distal-most urethra pierces the perineal membrane. The mucosa of the meatus is continuous with that of the vulva. Support of the urethra and bladder neck is believed to be important in the maintenance of continence during sudden increases in intra-abdominal pressure. The support mechanism is complex and incompletely understood.

The posterior wall of the urethra is embedded in and supported by the endopelvic connective tissue. This sheet of connective tissue consists of collagen, elastin, and a small amount of smooth muscle. The connective tissue envelops the anterior vagina. This supportive tissue has been likened to a sling or a hammock around the urethra and bladder neck.

The endopelvic connective tissue in this area is attached to the perineal membrane ventrally and laterally to the levator ani muscles by way of the arcus tendineus fascia pelvis (ATFP). The ATFP is a condensation of connective tissue, which extends bilaterally from the inferior part of the pubic bone along the junction of the fascia of the obturator internus and levator ani muscle group to an area near the ischial spine. This tissue provides secondary support to the urethra, bladder neck, and bladder base.

Defects in this tissue are believed to result in cystocele and urethral hypermobility. The primary support to this area and the entire pelvic floor is believed to be the levator ani muscles. At rest, the constant tone mediated by slow-twitch fibers constitutes the major supportive mechanism.

Fast-twitch fibers in these muscles cause the sudden stopping of the urinary stream to provide the voluntary guarding reflex. With acute increases in intra-abdominal pressure, forceful contraction of the fast-twitch levator fibers elevates the pelvic floor and tightens intact connective tissue planes, thereby supporting the pelvic viscera.

The anterior distal wall of the urethra is attached to the pubic bone by the pubourethral ligaments **(Figure 2.3)**. These ligaments consist of extensions of the perineal membrane and the caudal and ventral-most portion of the ATFP. The ligaments may limit movement of the anterior wall of the urethra during increases in intra-abdominal pressure but probably exert a lesser degree of support to the posterior wall.

The pubourethral ligaments suspend the female urethra under the pubic arch (**Figure 2.3**). The previously described endopelvic connective tissue, when intact, provides support to the urethra as a whole. With increases in intra-abdominal pressure, some believe that the urethra is compressed shut against this firm support.

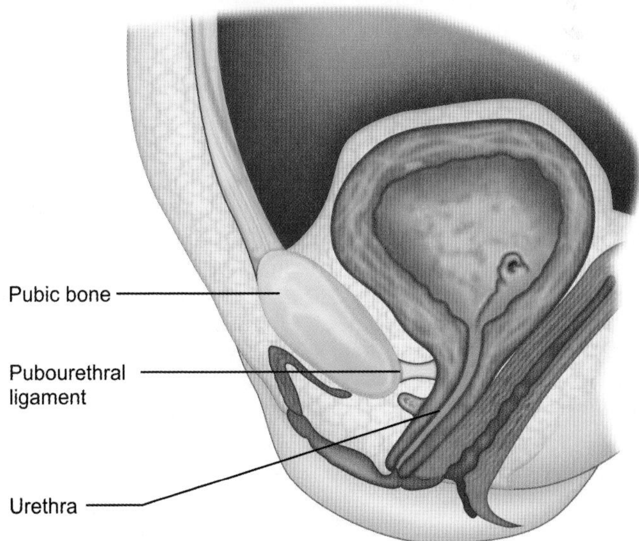

Figure 2.3: Pubourethral ligament

Deficiency in the hammock like support of the endopelvic connective tissue, coupled with relative preservation of the preferentially anterior urethral support of the pubourethral ligaments, may partially explain the complex rotational and descending motion of the bladder neck commonly observed in association with stress incontinence. The pubourethral ligaments may serve to limit downward motion of the anterior urethral wall and provide a pivot point for rotatory motion around the pubic bone.

Some theorize that this preferential anterior wall support also may serve to pull the anterior and posterior urethral walls apart during straining, thereby contributing to bladder neck incompetency and stress incontinence. Unlike male anatomy, in which the bladder neck and the prostate comprise the internal urinary sphincter, the internal sphincter in females is functional rather than anatomic. The bladder neck and proximal urethra constitute the female internal sphincter. The female external sphincter (i.e. the rhabdosphincter) has the most prominent effect on the female urethra at the urogenital triangle. Located approximately 1.8 cm distal to the bladder neck, it exerts influence for a distance of approximately 1.5 cm of urethral length.

The female urethra contains an internal sphincter and an external sphincter (**Figure 2.4**). The internal sphincter is more of a functional

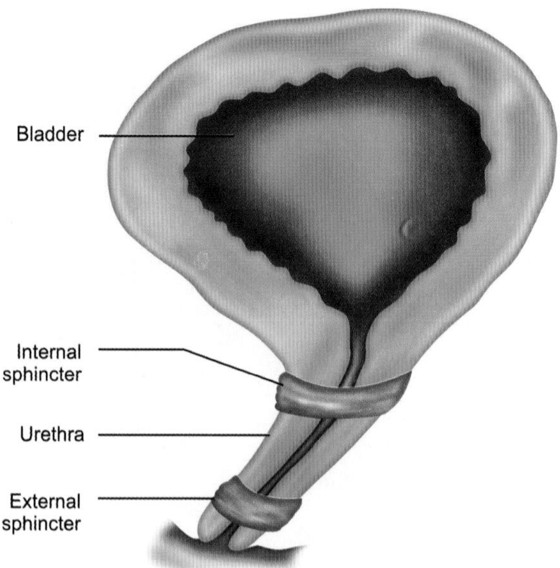

Figure 2.4: Urethral sphincters

concept than a distinct anatomic entity. The external sphincter is the muscle strengthened by Kegel exercises.

Bladder Anatomy (Figure 2.5)

The bladder wall is made up of muscle fibers extending in all directions. This configuration is well suited to decreasing the bladder size in all dimensions when contracting.

At the bladder neck, the muscular bladder wall is more organized, and three relatively distinct layers become apparent. The inner longitudinal layer fuses with the inner longitudinal layer of the urethra. The middle circular layer is most prominent in the proximity of the bladder neck, and it fuses with the deep trigonal muscle. The outer longitudinal layer contributes some anterior fibers to what become the pubovesical muscles, terminating on the posterior surface of the pubic bone.

These muscles may be important in bladder neck opening during micturition. Posteriorly, the outer longitudinal fibers interdigitate with deep trigonal fibers and the detrusor muscle. These fibers may aid in bladder neck closure.

The bladder mucosa is transitional epithelium, which is loosely connected to the muscular wall by way of a connective tissue layer

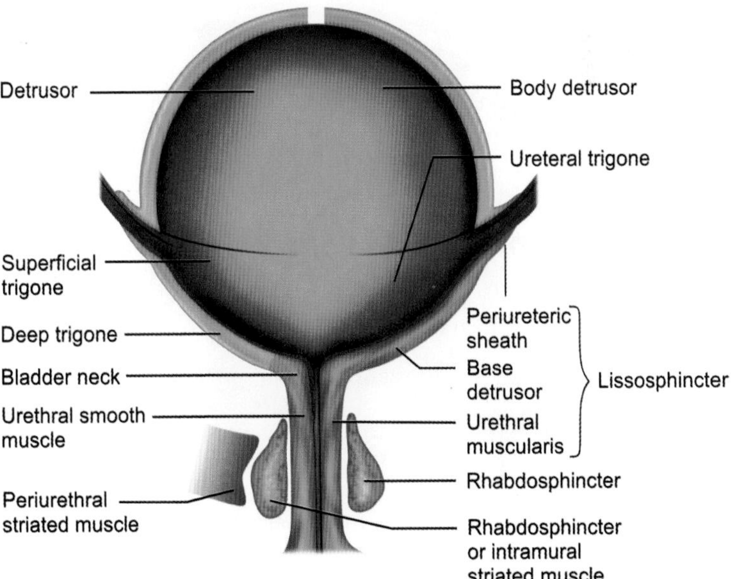

Figure 2.5: Bladder anatomy

called the lamina propria. At the trigone, the epithelium is more densely adherent to the underlying muscle.

The trigone is a triangular structure formed by the internal urethral opening and the orifices of the right and left ureter. The superior border of the trigone is a raised area called the interureteric ridge. Deep to the mucosa are two muscular layers. The superficial layer connects to longitudinal urethral musculature. The deep muscle fuses with detrusor and Waldeyer sheath, the fibromuscular covering of the intramural ureter. The intramural ureter enters the bladder wall obliquely. The muscle fibers are longitudinal in orientation at this point. This segment of the ureter is about 1.5 cm in length.

Retropubic Space Anatomy (Figure 2.6)

Ventrally, the retropubic space is bounded by the pubic bones and the midline fibrocartilage. The floor and part of the dorsal aspect consist of the bladder, urethra, and endopelvic connective tissue, which extend

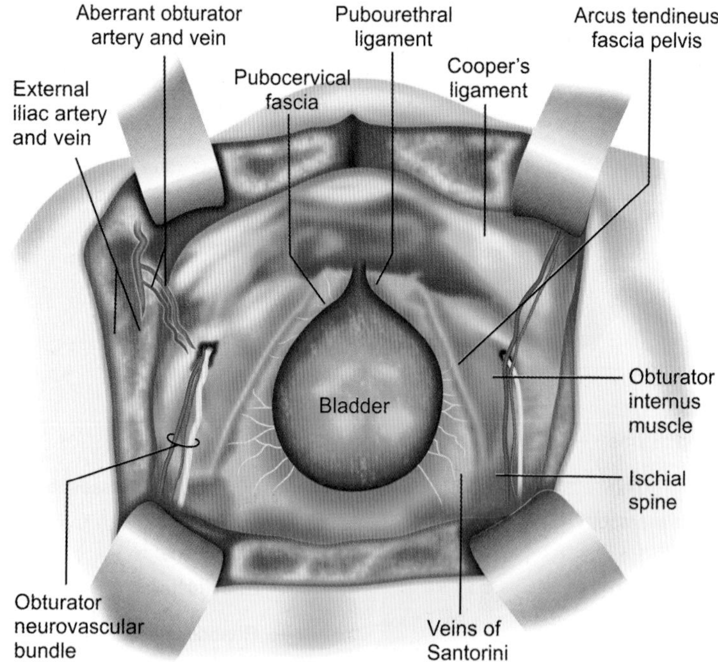

Figure 2.6: Retropubic space anatomy

laterally on both sides to the pelvic side walls at the arcus tendineus fascia pelvis (ATFP).

The remainder of the dorsal wall consists of the pelvic parietal peritoneum and the transversalis fascia. Above the arcuate line, the posterior rectus sheath is present. As originally described by Retzius, the potential space extends in a cephalad direction to the level of the umbilicus.[2]

The pectineal ligament or Cooper ligament, lies on the superior-dorsal surface of the pubic ramus. A flat triangular extension of Cooper ligament, the lacunar ligament, widens as it travels medially and joins the inguinal ligament at the pubic tubercle. The anterior or ventral aspect of the bladder makes up the floor of the retropubic space. This part of the bladder wall is extraperitoneal in location.

The cephalad wall and part of the posterior wall are covered with peritoneum and can be accessed from within the peritoneal cavity. The inferior aspect of the bladder lies on the anterior vagina, cervix, and lower uterine segment. The tissue between the bladder and the muscular wall of the vagina is the endopelvic connective tissue.

Lateral to the bladder and bladder neck and within the endopelvic connective tissue lies a venous plexus. These prominent veins are a frequent source of bleeding during retropubic urethropexy. The pubovesical ligaments, pubourethral ligaments, and extrinsic muscles of the urethra also lie in the retropubic space.

Pelvic Diaphragm Anatomy (Figure 2.7)

The pelvic diaphragm lines the floor of the bony pelvis and is composed of four sheets of muscles, the pubococcygeus, iliococcygeus, ischiococcygeus, and coccygeus.

The pelvic diaphragm (i.e. levator ani musculature) is composed of pubococcygeus, iliococcygeus, ischiococcygeus, and coccygeus muscles (**Figure 2.8**). It contains 3 openings through which the rectum, urethra, and cervix pass.

This is the side view of the pelvic diaphragm (**Figure 2.9**). The pelvic diaphragm supports the pelvic organs (e.g. bladder, uterus, and rectum).

Specialists often refer to the pelvic diaphragm as the levator ani. The levator ani musculature is attached to the inner sides of the bony pelvis by a condensation of pelvic fascia called the arcus tendineus.

The levator ani is the most important component of the pelvic diaphragm because the integrity of the pelvic floor depends upon its function. When the levator ani is damaged, stress urinary incontinence and/or herniation of pelvic organs through the vagina may develop.[3]

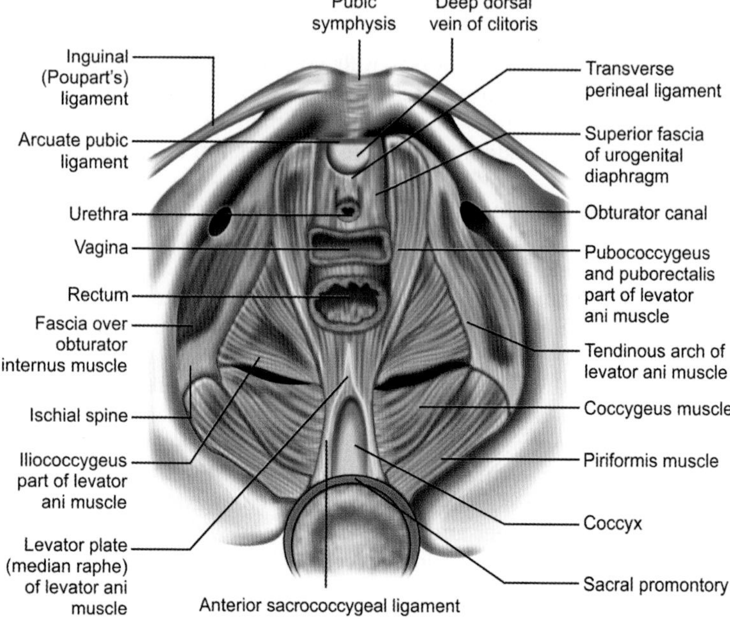

Figure 2.7: Superior view of pelvic diaphragm

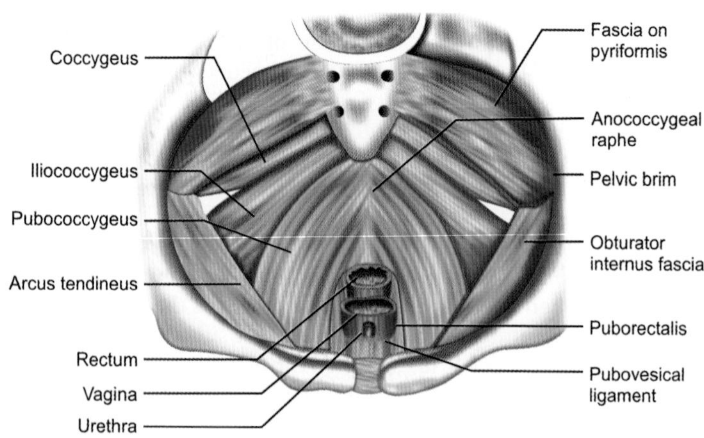

Figure 2.8: Levator ani muscle

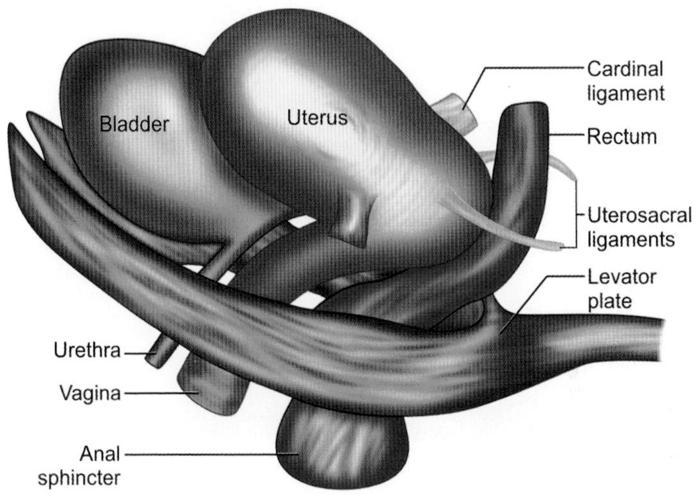

Figure 2.9: Side view of pelvic diaphragm

Transobturator Anatomy and Anatomy of the Inner Groin

The obturator membrane is a fibrous sheath that spans the obturator foramen, through which the obturator neurovascular bindle penetrates via the obturator canal (**Figure 2.10**). The obturator artery and vein originate as branches of internal iliac vessels.

As they emerge from the inferior side of the obturator membrane and enter the obturator space, they divide into many small branches supplying the muscles of the adductor compartment of the thigh. Obturator vessels are predominantly small (<5 mm in diameter) and splinter into variable courses. In contrast to the vessels, the obturator nerve emerges from the obturator membrane and bifurcates into anterior and posterior divisions traveling distally down the thigh to supply the muscles of the adductor compartment. With the patient in the dorsal lithotomy position, the nerves and vessels of the thigh course laterally away from the tissue of pubic ramus.

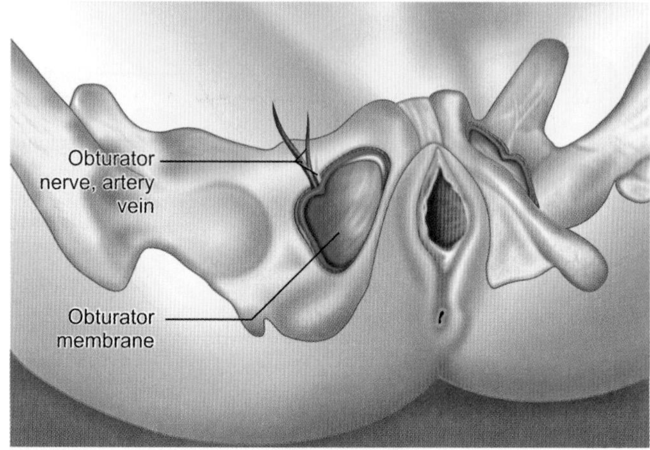

Figure 2.10: Anatomy of obturator membrane

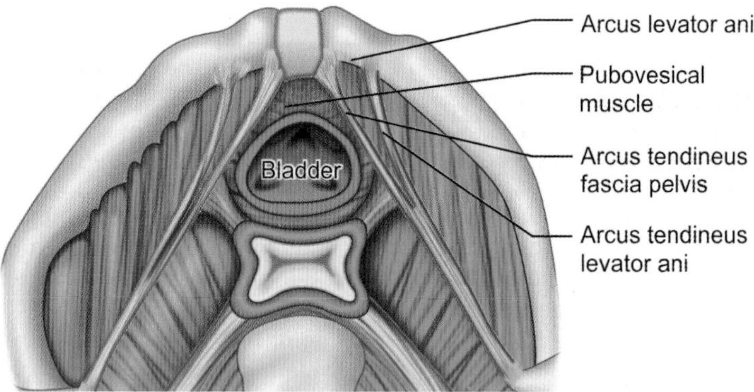

Figure 2.11: Supporting fascia

Supporting Ligaments and Fascia

The urethropelvic ligament is a fibrous band of connective tissue that lines the undersurface of the bladder neck and attaches laterally to the arcus tendineus (**Figure 2.11**). The urethropelvic ligament provides the major support to the bladder neck and proximal urethra. Laxity of the urethropelvic ligament results in stress urinary incontinence (SUI).

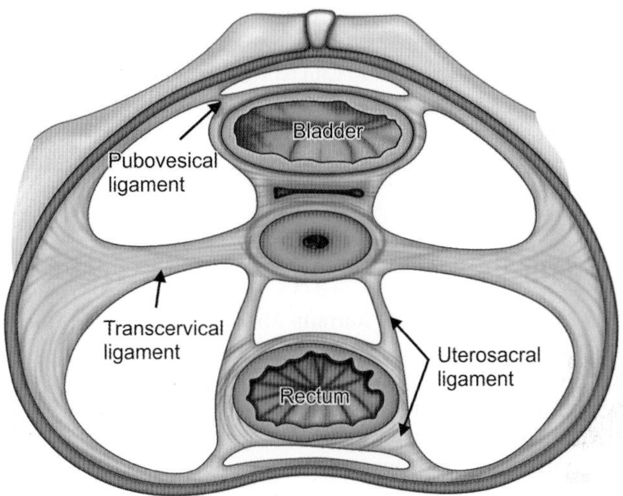

Figure 2.12: Supporting ligaments

The pubocervical fascia is a fibrous sheet of connective tissue that lines the base of the urinary bladder and inserts laterally into the arcus tendineus. An intact pubocervical fascia prevents the herniation of the bladder and the proximal urethra into the vagina. Damage to the pubocervical fascia may cause the bladder to herniate through the vagina, resulting in cystocele formation and SUI.

The cardinal ligaments arise from the arcus tendineus and anchor to the uterine cervix (**Figure 2.12**). The cardinal ligaments stabilize and support the uterus, vagina, and bladder. Weakening of the cardinal ligaments may cause a cystocele and uterine descent.

The uterosacral ligaments originate from condensation of the fibrous connective tissue overlying the sacral promontory and insert into the uterine cervix (**Figure 2.12**). The uterosacral ligaments stabilize the uterus in the bony pelvis. Weakening of the uterosacral ligaments may cause a prolapse uterus or vaginal vault prolapse.

References

1. Athanasiou S, Khullar V, Boos K, Salvatore S, Cardozo L. Imaging the urethral sphincter with three-dimensional ultrasound. Obstet Gynecol. 1999;94(2):295-301.

2. Kingsnorth AN, Skandalakis PN, Colborn GL, Weidman TA, Skandalakis LJ, Skandalakis JE. Embryology, anatomy, and surgical applications of the preperitoneal space. Surg Clin North Am. 2000;80(1):1-24.
3. Walters MD, Weber AM. Anatomy of the lower urinary tract, rectum and pelvic floor. In: Walters MD, Karram MM (Eds). Urogynecology and Pelvic Reconstructive Surgery. 2nd edn. St. Louis, Mo: Mosby; 2000.pp.3-13.

Bibliography

1. Brett J Vassallo, Mickey M Karram. Abdominal Operations for Urinary Stress Incontinence.
2. http://www.learnerhelp.com/pelvic%20diaphragm.html
3. life-tech/education/urology-education
4. medical-encyclopaedia/stress-incontinence
5. www.pelvicfloor.co.il/pages.asp.8

CHAPTER

3

Neuroanatomical Aspects of Lower Urinary Tract

Sandeep Patil, Sarika Dodwani, Prakash Trivedi

Intact neuroanatomy and neurophysiology are essential to both the storage and micturition phases of lower urinary tract function. These phases are controlled largely by the peripheral autonomic nervous system with important modulating information contributed by sensory nerves from the bladder and urethra. Further modification is provided by higher central nervous system (CNS) centers, which allow conscious control of lower urinary tract function. Lesions anywhere along these neuroanatomic pathways can contribute to or cause incontinence or voiding dysfunction.[1]

Voluntary control of detrusor activity is thought to arise in the frontal cerebral cortex (**Figure 3.1**). This area is in communication with the pontine mesencephalic reticular formation, which serves as the brainstem micturition center. Maturation of these and higher centers are important in the childhood acquisition of the ability to voluntarily suppress micturition. Diseases that involve this area of the brain may cause or contribute to incontinence disorders. Stroke, multiple sclerosis, Parkinson's disease, and brain tumors are examples.

Efferent connections beginning in the pons and terminating in the sacral micturition center at the S2 to S4 levels are important to efficient detrusor functioning during micturition. Damage to these tracts (e.g. spinal cord injury) results in detrusor areflexia. Neural activity within this system promotes micturition.

A neural loop involving the bladder, sacral micturition center, pontine micturition center, and urethral sphincter mechanism has been described. This pathway allows the coordination of urethral and detrusor function. In other words, coordination of urethral relaxation with detrusor contraction is dependent on this neural pathway being intact.

Dysfunction in this loop may result in detrusor-sphincter dyssynergia. Direct connections between the cerebral cortex and the sacral-pudendal

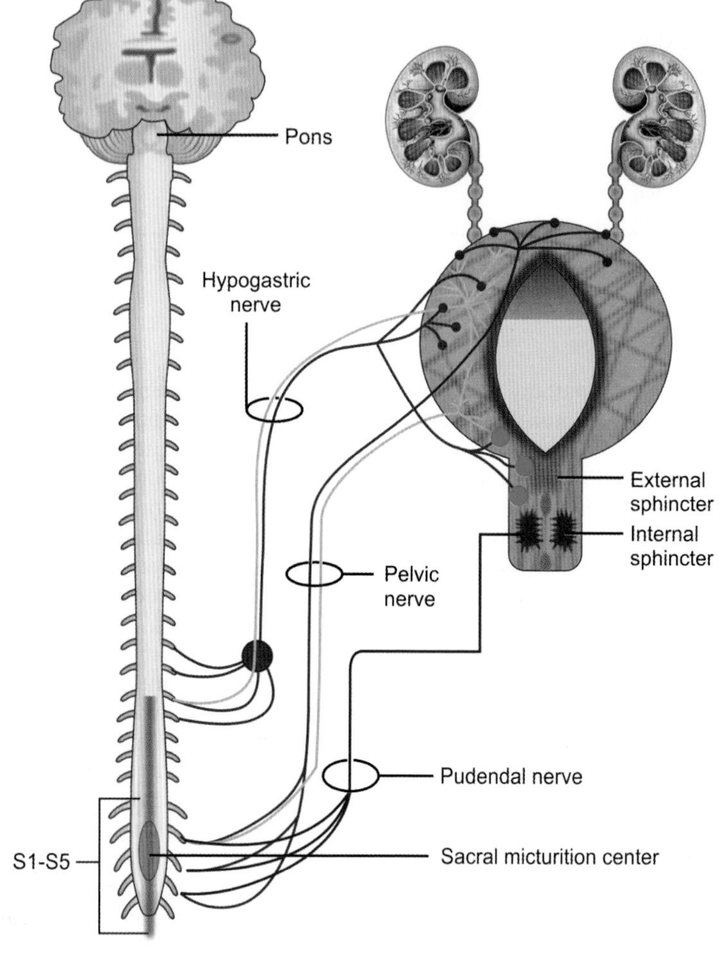

Figure 3.1: CNS control of micturition

motor neurons are important contributors to voluntary control over the striated urethral-sphincter complex. Severe neuromuscular damage to the striated urethral muscles, along with brain and spinal cord injury, can prevent proper functioning of this system.[2]

Healthy functioning of the lower urinary tract is partly dependent on the interplay of sympathetic (i.e. adrenergic) and parasympathetic (i.e. cholinergic) input to the bladder and urethra (**Figure 3.2**). Bladder filling normally takes place with little or no increase in intravesical pressure.

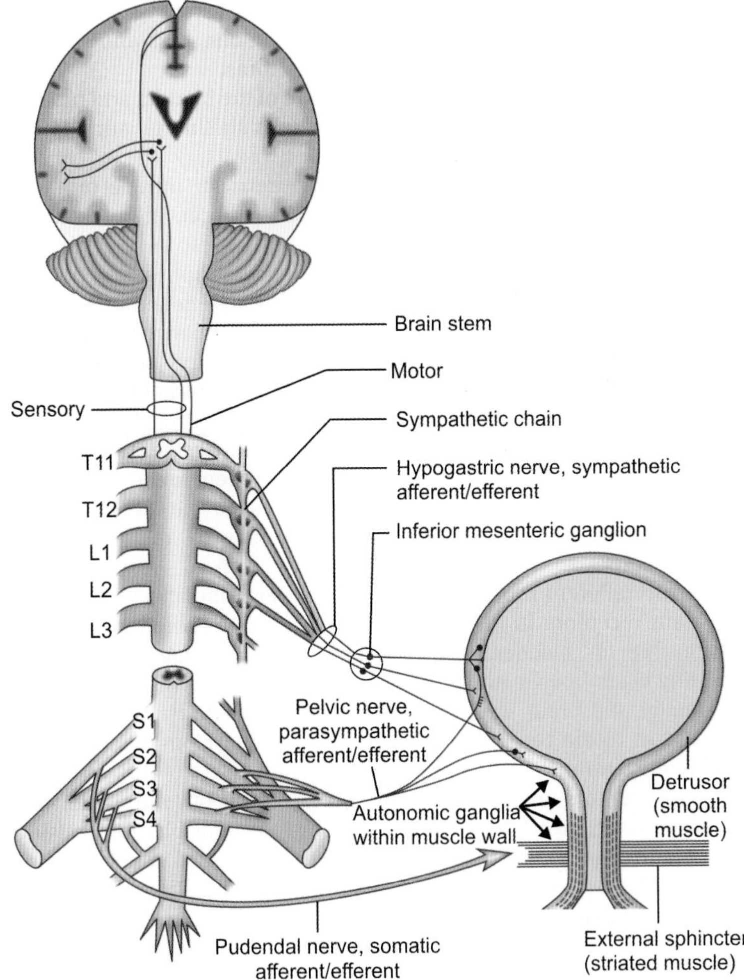

Figure 3.2: Autonomic nervous system control of micturition

This phenomenon is largely due to the predominance of sympathetic tone during the filling and storage phase. Simplistically, beta-adrenergic receptors predominate in the detrusor muscle.

Stimulation of these receptors promotes bladder relaxation. Alpha fibers also exist, in smaller numbers, in the parasympathetic ganglia supplying the bladder. Stimulation of the alpha fibers results in the inhibition of neural firing at the level of the parasympathetic ganglion, thereby inhibiting bladder contractions. Alpha-adrenergic receptors predominate in the smooth muscle of the bladder, neck and urethra. Stimulation results in contraction of the structures.

The sum effect of sympathetic stimulation of the bladder and urethra is the promotion of storage. Parasympathetic or cholinergic stimulation generally is micturition-promoting.

Postganglionic muscarinic fibers to the detrusor muscle promote bladder contractions when stimulated. In addition, stimulation of muscarinic receptors on alpha-adrenergic nerves to the urethra prevents norepinephrine stimulation. The resulting physiologic effect is urethral relaxation. Cholinergic agents, although generally thought of as promoters of detrusor activity, also can stimulate preganglionic sympathetic nicotinic receptors with neural connections to the urethra and bladder neck. Such stimulation promotes contraction of these structures.

Nonadrenergic, noncholinergic nerves with adenosine triphosphate (ATP)—stimulated purinergic receptors have been found in animal models and in the human bladder. These nerves may be very important in bladder contractility. Prostaglandins also may be able to activate these receptors.

Sensory afferent innervation of the bladder originates with stretch and pain receptors in the bladder wall. Stretch receptors, which are responsible for bladder proprioception, are the origin of impulses traveling via the pelvic nerve to the posterior columns ipsilaterally and eventually, the brain stem micturition center. Connections from the brain stem to the cerebral cortex provide for conscious awareness of bladder distention.

Pain receptors are present in the bladder wall but not as densely as stretch receptors. These receptors are responsible for sensing temperature, touch, and irritative stimuli. The generated impulses travel by way of the hypogastric nerve to synapse in the posterior root ganglia. The impulses cross to the contralateral side before ascending in the spinothalamic tract and the thalamic nuclei, eventually reaching the cerebral cortex.

Afferent impulses from these pain receptors can trigger detrusor contractions via a normally suppressed reflex arc. Under conditions of severe mucosal irritation (e.g. urinary tract infection), this reflex may become unmasked. In addition, disorders resulting in the loss of conscious cerebral cortical input may be responsible for the emergence of this reflex.

Somatic efferent innervation to the striated urethral sphincter complex is from the second through the fourth sacral segments. The precise source of these fibers is controversial. Evidence suggests that the sphincter complex is innervated by way of the pelvic nerve rather than the pudendal nerve, as was once thought. The levator ani complex probably has a dual source of innervation from both the pelvic and pudendal nerves.

In women, estrogen receptors can be found in the musculature of the pelvic floor, bladder, bladder neck, and urethra. Estrogen stimulation increases the density of alpha-adrenergic receptors in the urethral smooth muscle. Progesterone may enhance beta-adrenergic activity. Emerging evidence of the presence of gonadotropin receptors in the lower urinary tract also exists.[3]

References

1. Clemens JQ. Basic bladder neurophysiology. Urol Clin North Am. 2010;37(4):487-94. doi: 10.1016.
2. Chai TC, Steers WD. Neurophysiology of micturition and continence in women. Int Urogynecol J Pelvic Floor Dysfunct. 1997;8(2):85-97.
3. Yoshimura N, Miyazato M. Neurophysiology and therapeutic receptor targets for stress urinary incontinence. Int J Urol. 2012;19(6):524-37.

CHAPTER

4

Evaluation of a Patient Prior to Treatment of Urinary Incontinence and Role of Urodynamics

Amita Jain

Urinary incontinence (UI) is a common symptom that can affect women of all ages, with a wide range of severity and nature. Hence extent and interpretation of its evaluation must be tailored to the individual need. Urinary incontinence patients have to be approached with a defined protocol. Focus should be on identifying the type of incontinence, understanding the effect of the condition on the patients' quality of life and her expectations from the treatment, identifying associated problems, and thorough and effective counseling so that a consensus is met as regards the treatment to be planned. The aim of this chapter is to provide sensible and practical guidance for planning and designing management of UI rather than an exhaustive narrative review.

History Taking and Physical Examination

The clinical assessment of any ailment starts with history taking. The presenting symptoms should be explored for minor details like duration, most bothersome one, frequency, precipitants, etc. This helps in categorizing the patient's UI as stress urinary incontinence (SUI), urge urinary incontinence (UUI)/overactive bladder (OAB) syndrome, mixed urinary incontinence (MUI), or overflow urinary incontinence (**Table 4.1**).

National Institute for Health and Clinical Excellence (NICE) recommends that initial treatment should be started on this basis. In MUI, treatment should be directed towards the predominant symptom [Grade D: Body of evidence is weak and recommendation must be applied with caution: Good Practice Point (D GPP)].[1]

According to European Association of Urology (EAU), initial assessment should also include a medical, neurological, obstetric and gynecological history; which may help to understand the underlying cause and identify factors that may impact on treatment decisions. The patient should also be asked about previous pelvic surgeries or any

Table 4.1: Categorizing of patients of UI on basis of symptoms

	Questions	*Stress UI*	*Urge UI*	*Overflow UI*
1.	Description of incontinent episodes	Loss with activity, cough	Sudden urgency; inability to reach toilet	Continuous slow loss
2.	Precipitating factors	Cough, physical activity	Full bladder, sensory triggers	None, stress may worsen
3.	Urinary frequency	Normal	Increased	Hesitancy; inability to void
4.	Nocturia	<1	Variable	Nocturnal enuresis
5.	Volume loss	Small	Large	Continuous

comorbid conditions and also details of current medications, whether taken for her urinary problem or some other indications. Symptoms of pelvic organ prolapse, defecatory dysfunction, pelvic pain and sexual dysfunction should also be sought. Again these may have impact on symptoms of UI, or may cause it [Grade A].[2]

Physical examination of a patient with UI should include general examination to assess edema, neurologic abnormalities, mobility, cognition, dexterity; abdominal examination, to detect an enlarged bladder or other abdominal mass, and perineal and digital examination of the rectum and/or vagina. Examining the perineum includes a careful assessment of estrogen status and any associated genitourinary prolapse.

A Cough Stress Test

Provocative test for SUI can confirm presence of the sign of SUI and usually done with cough or provocative stress test. The cough stress test can be performed with bladder empty or filled and with the patient supine or standing. For the test patient is asked to cough vigorously several times while the examiner observes for the urine loss from the meatus. Any leakage of urine with provocation is considered positive test.

Ideally the bladder is filled up to 300 mL or to a sense of fullness. However the test can also be performed with a empty bladder. In the supine empty stress test the patient voids immediately before examination in the lithotomy position and coughs or strains while the examiner inspects the urethral meatus. In either the full or the empty test if leakage does not occur in the supine lithotomy position patient repeats the maneuvers in the standing position and semiflexed knees in standing position. Some studies have corelated a positive empty supine stress test with objective urodynamics testing indicative of intrinsic sphincter deficiency.

Hypermobility

Some debate surrounds the roll of urethral hypermobility or lack thereof in the assessment of SUI. Urethral hypermobility refers to the degree of rotation and descent of urethra away from its retropubic position with increased abdominal pressure and these considered a sign of loss of urethral support. When urine leakage occurs without urethral hypermobility intrinsic sphincter deficiency is suspected.

The cotton tipped swab (Q-tip) test (**Figure 4.1**) was designed to quantify the degree of hypermobility by measuring the angle of deflection from horizontal of the swab inserted into the urethra during cough or Valsalva maneuver. To perform the test a swab is inserted per urethra to the level of the urethrovesical junction and the angle of swab compared with the horizontal is at rest. Next the patient cough's or strains and the change in the angle of swab is noted. An excursion 30 degrees or more of the tip outer tip upwards is positive test for hypermobility. Although this test is not a diagnostic test it is an objective measure.

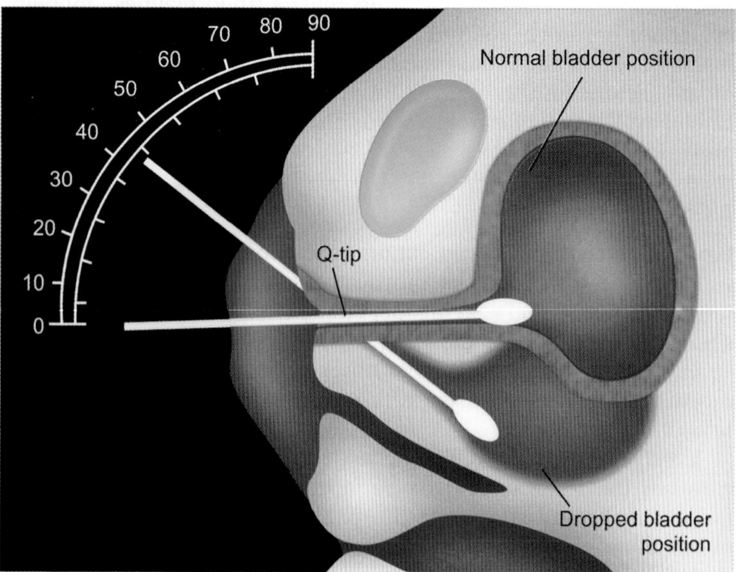

Figure 4.1: Q-tip test

Pelvic Organ Prolapse

The degree of pelvic organ prolapse (POP) should be described using common grading and staging methods. The two most common methods include the POP quantification and Baden-Walker systems. Both methods attempt to standardize the description and the degree of pelvic organ descent, using the hymen as a fixed point of reference.

Pelvic floor assessment: It is integral to continence and is done by means of digital vaginal examination. Two fingers are kept posteriorly in the vagina at 2 to 4 cm from the hymenal ring and patient is asked to contract the muscles as used to "hold their urine" or "to avoid passing gas". Her ability to contract pelvic muscles of each side with their strength and duration of contraction is judged and graded.

National Institute for Health and Clinical Excellence (NICE) stats poor inter- and intraobserver reliability of grading systems [EL = 3], however recommends routine digital assessment of pelvic floor muscle contraction before the use of supervised pelvic floor muscle training for the treatment of UI [D (GPP)].[1]

Referral

The clinical assessment should seek to identify relevant predisposing and precipitating factors and other diagnoses that may require referral for additional investigation and treatment. According to NICE, conditions that need an urgent referral are microscopic hematuria in women aged 50 years and older, visible hematuria, recurrent or persisting urinary tract infection (UTI) associated with hematuria in women aged 40 years and older and suspected malignant mass arising from the urinary tract. In addition, symptomatic prolapse that is visible at or below the vaginal introitus or the finding of a palpable bladder on bimanual or abdominal examination after voiding should also be referred for further management [D (GPP)].[1]

Referral to a specialist service should be considered in presence of persisting bladder or urethral pain, clinically benign pelvic masses, associated fecal incontinence, suspected neurological disease, symptoms of voiding difficulty, suspected urogenital fistulae and; with past history of continence surgery, pelvic cancer surgery or pelvic radiation therapy[1] [GR A].[2]

Patient Questionnaires

Assessment of impact on quality of life (QoL) should also be done by finding out the alteration in lifestyle like use of pads or other measures to hide urine leakage. The NICE has recommended International

Consultation on Incontinence Questionnaire (ICIQ), the Bristol Female Lower Urinary Tract Symptoms Questionnaire (BFLUTS), Incontinence QoL Questionnaire (I-QoL), Stress and Urge Incontinence and Quality of Life Questionnaire (SUIQQ), Urinary Incontinence Severity Score (UISS) Stress-related leak, Emptying ability, Anatomy, Protection, Inhibition, Quality of life, Mobility and Mental Status Incontinence Classification System (SEAPI-QMM), Incontinence Severity Score (ISI), the King's Health Questionnaire for evaluation of therapies as the test—retest reliability of these is good [D (GPP)].[1] But EAU has cautioned health care professionals to be aware that the use of questionnaires and patient-reported outcome measures has not been shown to influence patient outcome in UI due to the lack of specific research in this area [GR C].[2]

Voiding Diaries

Voiding diaries are a semiobjective method of quantifying symptoms, such as daytime and night-time frequency, urgency, UUI and SUI episodes. They also quantify urodynamic variables, such as voided volume and 24-hour or nocturnal total urine volume.

Commonly used voiding diaries are micturition time charts, frequency/volume charts and bladder diaries. Micturition time charts record only the times of micturitions for a minimum of 24 continuous hours. Frequency volume charts record voided volumes in addition with times of micturitions for a minimum of 24-hour and bladder diaries also include information on incontinence episodes, pad usage, fluid intake, degree of urgency and degree of incontinence.

Normal voiding frequency varies between 5 and 8 times per 24 hours in women, where frequency increases in women of older age, with a mean of 6.9 in the third decade and 8.2 in the sixth decade. Total urine volume per day fluctuates between 1,350 and 1,800 mL; while mean voided volume (VV) ranges approximately between 200 and 250 mL.[3] However, the International Continence Society (ICS) definition of daytime frequency is when the patient considers that he/she is voiding too often.[4] No absolute number can still be applied to define a cut-off value for voiding frequency.

Any discrepancy between diary recordings and the patient rating of symptoms, e.g. frequency or UI, can be useful in patient management. In addition, voided volume measurement can be used to support diagnoses, such OAB or polyuria. Diaries can also be used to monitor treatment response.

European Association of Urology recommends voiding diaries of 3 to 7 days duration to evaluate coexisting storage and voiding dysfunction in clinical practice and in research [GR A].[2] NICE also recommends use of bladder diaries for initial assessment of women with UI or OAB and states that women should be encouraged to complete a minimum of 3 days of the diary covering variations in their usual activities, such as both working and leisure days [D (GPP)].[1]

Pad Test

The simplest method of measuring urine loss, by weighing a perineal pad before and after use, was described by Caldwell in 1974.[5] The pad test is a diagnostic tool that assesses the degree of incontinence in patients in a semiobjective manner.

Short-term (1-Hour) Pad Test

It is often used in office practice because of its convenient nature. Patient is asked to drink a fixed amount of fluid (500 mL of sodium-free liquid) within 15 minutes. Specific standardized physical activities are performed in 1-hour time, including walking, climbing stairs, standing, coughing vigorously, running on the spot, bending to pick up objects, and hand washing with running water. After 1 hour, any increment in pad weight of more than 1 g is considered incontinence.

Long-term Pad Test

It requires patients to wear pads for 24 or 48 hours during regular everyday activities. Patients are instructed to record the frequency and amount of fluid intake as well as their episodes of micturition and incontinence. The pad is weighed at the end of the test. Pads are collected in resealed plastic bags. Incontinence is diagnosed if pad weight is more than 8 g/24 hours on the long-term pad test.[3]

Although the ICS has attempted to standardize pad testing, there remains variation in the duration of the test and the physical activity undertaken during the test. The subjective assessment of incontinence is difficult to interpret and may not indicate reliably the degree of abnormality. A pad test cannot differentiate between causes of UI. Other drawbacks are chances of false-positive results due to perspiration and vaginal discharge and false-negative results due to drying out. Patient adherence to home pad testing protocols is poor and there could be a problem of weighing scale accuracy.

Pad tests are not recommended by NICE in the routine assessment of women with UI [D].[1] While EAU recommends use of pad test for quantification of UI and use of repeat pad test to measure objective treatment outcome [GR C], but also states that home-based pad tests longer than 24 hours provide no additional benefit and a weight gain > 1.3 g in a 24-hour home-based test can be used as a diagnostic threshold for UI.[2]

Urinalysis

Simple reagent strip ('dipstick') urinalysis can provide useful screening information in women with UI. Presence of nitrite and leukocyte esterase may indicate UTI. Proteins are suggestive of infection and/or renal disease. In presence of blood, malignancy (or infection) should be ruled out and glucose in urine indicates uncontrolled diabetes mellitus. These all conditions may be associated with symptoms of OAB. Especially UI is known to occur more commonly in women with urinary tract infections (UTIs) and is also more likely in the first few days following an acute infection.[6] In contrast with symptomatic UTI, asymptomatic bacteriuria appears to have little influence on UI.

National Institute for Health and Clinical Excellence (NICE) recommends use of urine dipstick tests in all women presenting with UI to detect blood, glucose, protein, leukocytes and nitrites [D (GPP)].[1] EAU also recommends urinalysis as a part of the initial assessment of a patient with UI and suggest that treat symptomatic UTI appropriately, but do not treat asymptomatic bacteriuria in elderly patients to improve urinary incontinence [GR A].[2] A study carried out in nursing home residents showed that the severity of UI was unchanged after eradication of bacteriuria.[7]

Microscopy and other tests may be necessary to confirm any abnormalities identified on dipstick analysis.

Postvoiding Residual Volume

Postvoiding residual (PVR) volume is the amount of urine that remains in the bladder after voiding. It indicates poor voiding efficiency, which may result from a number of contributing factors. Both bladder outlet obstruction and detrusor underactivity contribute to the development of PVR. It is important because it may worsen symptoms and, more rarely, may be associated with upper urinary tract dilatation and renal insufficiency.

Postvoiding residual can be measured by catheterization or ultrasound (USG). The results of studies investigating the best method of measuring PVR have led to the consensus that USG measurement of PVR (bladder scan) is better than measurement using catheterization.[8-13] The former is less invasive with fewer adverse effects. The NICE recommends bladder scan in preference to catheterization [D (GPP)], in women with symptoms suggestive of voiding dysfunction or recurrent UTI [B (DS)].[1] However, portable office ultrasound bladder scanners have a measure of operator independence and can be inaccurate in several clinical circumstances including obesity, prior lower abdominal surgery, cystic pelvic pathology, pregnancy, peritoneal dialysis and in the setting of ascites.[14]

EAU recommends measurement of PVR by USG [GR A], in patients with UI who have voiding dysfunction or who are receiving treatments that may cause or worsen voiding dysfunction [GR B] and when assessing patients with complicated UI [GR C].[2] Common Indications in clinical practice are symptoms of incomplete emptying, longstanding diabetes mellitus, history of urinary retention, failure of pharmacologic therapy, presence of pelvic floor prolapse and history of previous incontinence surgery.

The prevalence of PVR is uncertain, partly because of the lack of a standard definition of an abnormal PVR volume. In one recent prospective study the incidence of a PVR ≥ 100 mL, after one spontaneous void was 14 percent among symptomatic women, which is declined to 1.3 percent after repeated measurements. Voided volumes did not vary between voids. A falsely elevated PVR may result from rapid diuresis or psychogenic inhibition (for example patient difficulty with emptying due to environmental factors), amongst other factors. Therefore a single PVR measurement ≥100 mL is unreliable and needs repetition to confirm consistency before firm conclusions are drawn.[15]

Imaging

Imaging improves our understanding of the anatomical and functional abnormalities that may cause UI. Magnetic resonance imaging (MRI) provides good global pelvic floor assessment, including pelvic organ prolapse, defecatory function and integrity of the pelvic floor support structure.[16] The USG is preferred to MRI because of its ability to produce three-dimensional and four-dimensional (dynamic) images at lower cost and wider availability.

Several imaging studies have investigated the relationship between sphincter volume and function in women,[17] a particular pattern of urethrovesical movements to diagnose UI,[18] association of increased urethral mobility after childbirth to *de novo* SUI[19] and to assess the effect of sling insertion for SUI on midurethra.[20,21]

However, imaging (MRI, computed tomography, X-ray) is not recommended by NICE for the routine assessment of women with UI. The USG is recommended only for the assessment of PVR.[1] EAU also do not recommend routine imaging of the upper or lower urinary tract as part of the assessment of uncomplicated SUI in women.[2]

Other Tests

Bonney, Marshall and Fluid-Bridge tests are not recommended by NICE for assessment of women with UI [D]. Cystoscopy is not recommended in the initial assessment [D (GPP)] and should only be considered in case of reduced bladder capacity; suspected urethrovaginal/vesicovaginal fistula, interstitial cystitis or neoplasm.[1]

Urodynamics

This test is designed to determine the functional status of the bladder and urethra. In clinical practice, it is generally used as a collective term for all tests of bladder and urethral function. This includes both noninvasive estimation of urine flow, i.e. uroflowmetry; and invasive tests including multichannel cystometry, ambulatory monitoring and videourodynamics; and different tests of urethral function, such as urethral pressure profilometry, Valsalva leak point pressure estimation and retrograde urethral resistance measurement.

Uroflowmetry

Uroflowmetry entails a free-flow void into a recording device, which provides the practitioner with information about the volume of urine passed, the maximum (Q_{max}) and average rate of urine flow (Q_{ave}), voiding time, flow time and time to maximum flow[22] **(Figures 4.2 to 4.4).**[23] Q_{ave} in women usually ranges from 17 to 24 mL/s and Q_{max} from 23 to 33 mL/s. Voided volume (VV) varies between 250 and 550 mL.[3]

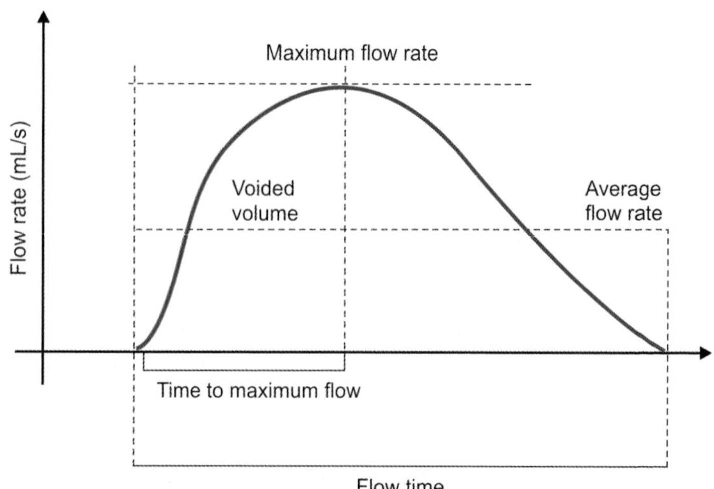

Figure 4.2: Normal bell-shaped flow curve of flow rate versus time[22]

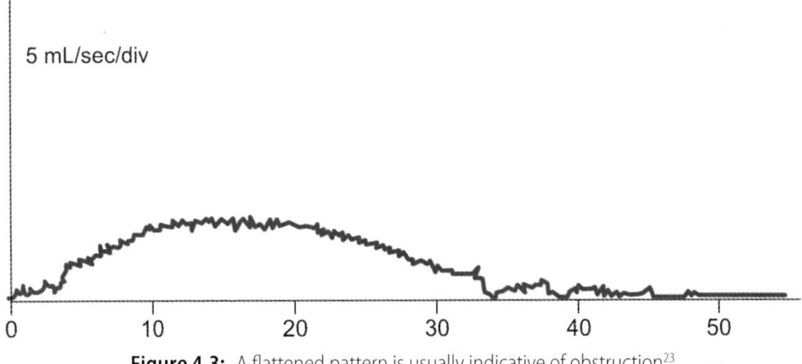

Figure 4.3: A flattened pattern is usually indicative of obstruction[23]

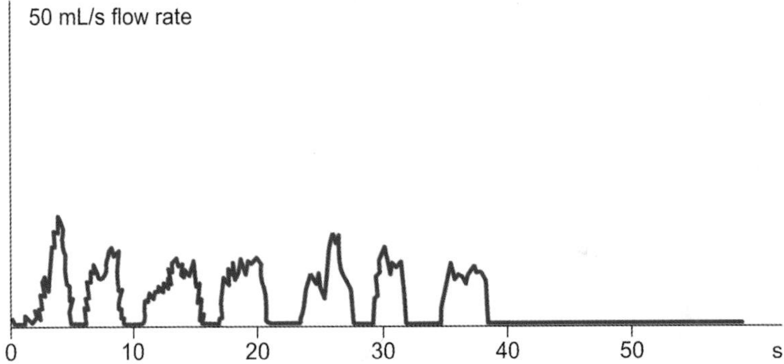

Figure 4.4: An interrupted or straining pattern, which can be seen with impaired bladder contractility, obstruction, or voiding with or by abdominal straining[23]

Pressure Flow Studies: Voiding Cystometry

This involves the measurement of detrusor pressure during controlled bladder filling and subsequent voiding with measurement of flow rate. Measurement of intravesical pressure can be carried out through a single recording channel called simple cystometry or, more commonly, by multichannel cystometry, which involves the synchronous measurement of both bladder and intra-abdominal pressures by means of catheters inserted into the bladder and the rectum or vagina (**Figure 4.5**). The aim is to replicate the woman's symptoms by filling the bladder and observing pressures changes or leakage caused by provocation tests (**Table 4.2**)[3] (**Figure 4.6**).[24]

There are some practical points to be taken care of while doing this test. Patient should be in favorable surroundings and should not be unduly stressed. Pressure flow studies (PFS) should be deferred for

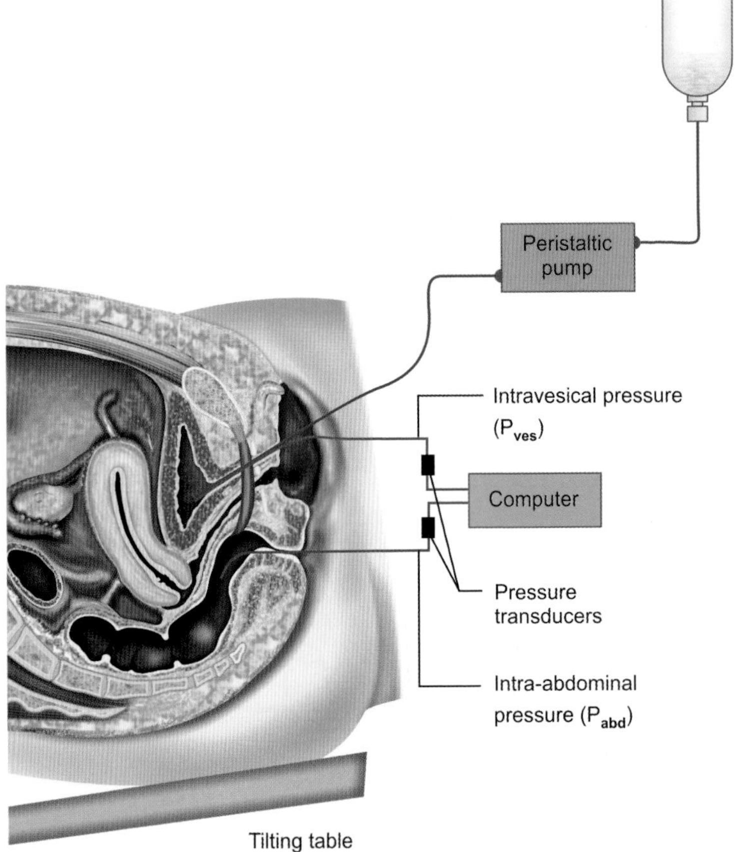

Figure 4.5: Catheter positions. Patient is supine only for catheter insertion (From Textbook of Female Urology and Urogynecology by Cardozo and Staskin, Second Edition)

appropriate time; if there is indwelling catheter (ideally catheter should be removed and instead clean intermittent self-catheterization should be started), UTI, history of recent instrumentation, for example cystoscopy, or recent medication impacting bladder function has been taken. Though routine prophylactic antibiotics are not needed for this test, but in case of high-risk patients (cardiac valve, orthopedic prosthesis, GU prosthesis, pacemakers) parental antibiotic prophylaxis might be necessary.

Videourodynamics

This PFS involves use of contrast medium instead of saline, to assess position and mobility of bladder neck in addition. Though it is expensive

Table 4.2: Normal urodynamic parameters in women[3]	
Filling phase	
Maximum bladder capacity: 450	450–550 mL
Normal first sensation: 100	100–250 mL
Bladder compliance: 30	30–100 mL/cm H_2O
Detrusor pressure (P_{det})	<6–10 cm H_2O*
Voiding phase	
Voided volume	250–650 mL
Q_{max}	13–25 mL/s
P_{det}@Q_{max}	18–30 cm H_2O
P_{det}@opening	22–46 cm H_2O

*Constantly low pressure that usually does not reach more than 6–10 cm H_2O above baseline at the end of filling (end-filling pressure) and there should be no involuntary contractions.

and involves radiation, but useful where anatomic structure and function are important for diagnosis and equivocal results from other tests.

Ambulatory Urodynamics

Ambulatory urodynamic studies are defined as a functional test of the lower urinary tract, using natural filling and reproducing the subject's everyday activities. It is done, when conventional urodynamic investigation may be unsuitable or fails to reproduce or explain LUTS as in neurogenic lower urinary tract dysfunction.

Electromyography of the pelvic floor and external urethral sphincter: Electromyography (EMG) activity increases progressively during bladder filling. The rise in electromyography activity during heightened abdominal pressure (cough, straining, etc.) is proportional to the level of stress. EMG activity of the external sphincter and pelvic muscles should be silent during voiding.[3]

Urethral Pressure Studies[3] (Table 4.3)

Leak Point Pressures

Detrusor leak point pressure (DLPP) is defined by the ICS as the lowest detrusor pressure at which urine leakage occurs in absence of either detrusor contraction or increased abdominal pressure.[26]

Abdominal leak point pressure (ALPP) or Valsalva leak point pressure (VLPP) is a measurement of urethral function or outlet competence

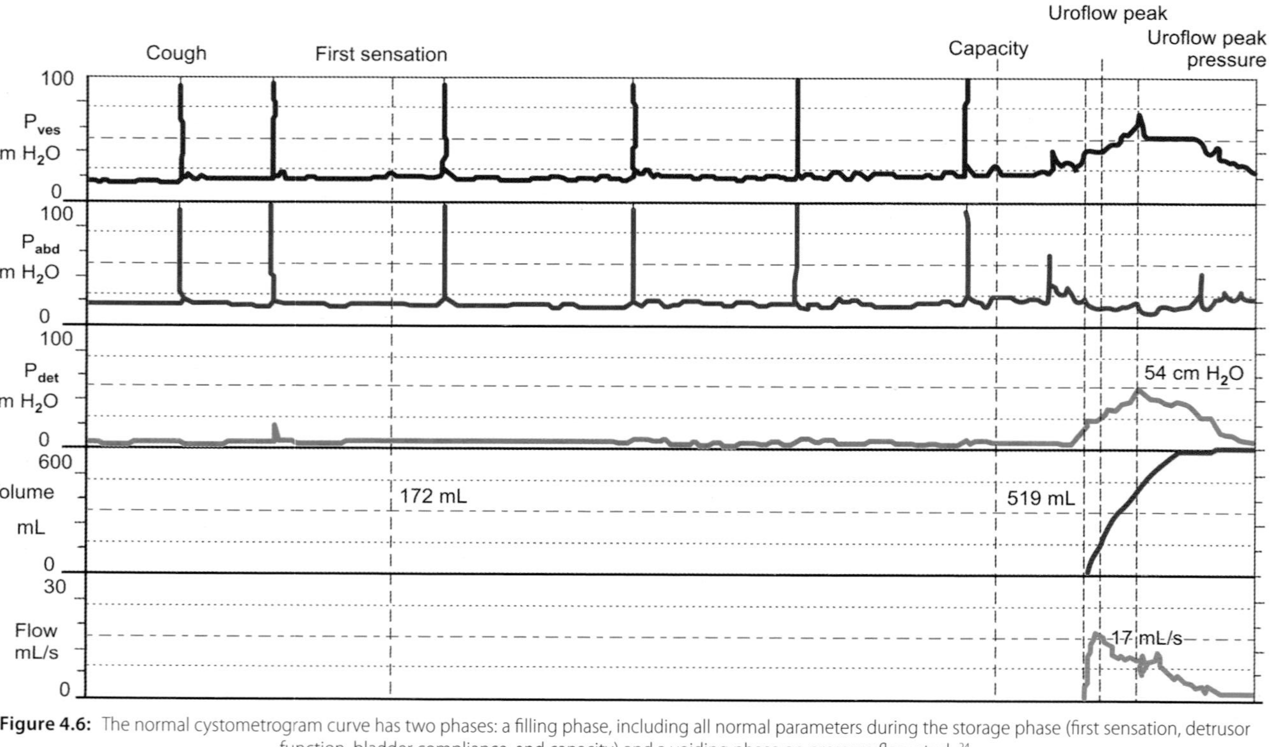

Figure 4.6: The normal cystometrogram curve has two phases: a filling phase, including all normal parameters during the storage phase (first sensation, detrusor function, bladder compliance, and capacity) and a voiding phase on pressure flow study[24]

Table 4.3: Diagnosis in patients of UI on basis of urethral pressure studies[3]

In neurogenic patients	
DLPP > 40 cm H_2O	Dangerous for the upper tract
In women with SUI	
VLPP < 60 cm H_2O	ISD (Intrinsic sphincter deficiency)
VLPP ≥100 cm H_2O	Urethral hypermobility
VLPP between 60 and 100 cm H_2O	Both ISD and hypermobility
MUCP < 20 cm H_2O	ISD
MUCP > 75 cm H_2O	Hypertonic

Notes:

1. There should be no 'DLPP/VLPP' in normal individuals
2. Patients with high grade cystocele may have a high LPP but MUCP remains low in existence of ISD.

and is the intravesical pressure at which urine leakage occurs due to increased abdominal pressure in the absence of a detrusor contraction.[14]

Urethral Pressure Profilometry

Urethral pressure profilometry (UPP) is the continuous fluid pressure needed to just open a closed urethra,[14] maximum urethral pressure (MUP) is categorized as maximum pressure of the measured profile, while maximum urethral closure pressure (MUCP) is defined as the maximum difference between urethral pressure and intravesical pressure.

Discussion

There is a low level of agreement between diagnostic value of history taking and urodynamic findings [LE 3].[2] However, generally women who do not report mixed or urge UI are unlikely to have findings of MUI or detrusor overactivity (DO) on urodynamics [EL = DS III].[1] But few studies have shown that around 20 percent patients without complaints of OAB may show DO on urodynamics.[25]

A recently published study on 55 women with SUI showed agreement between urodynamics and cough stress test in 89 percent of women (k = 0.51), between urodynamics and pad test in 60 percent (k = 0.08) and between stress test and pad test in 67 percent (k = 0.26). They concluded that cough stress test is more reliable than pad test for documentation of SUI.[26]

Previous work in women with UI has shown that 50 to 74 percent of patients with MUI see improvement in the UUI component after anti-incontinence surgery.[27] Mean DOLPP in subjective MUI was found to be less than pure UUI ($p = 0.004$) and P_{det}@Qmax was lower in the DO leakage group versus DO alone ($p = 0.05$) likely reflecting outlet resistance. This again suggests that increasing outlet resistance may improve symptoms of UUI.[28] On the other hand, there are some fallacies of MUCP, as it can be augmented voluntarily by 20 percent of symptomatic patients[29] and it decreases with age.[30] Therefore EAU do not recommend a routine urethral pressure profilometry [GR C].[2]

Recently an E-survey was done on 260 targeted Dutch specialists (gynecologists and urologists). Out of 163 (63%) respondents, 37 percent chose to perform standard preoperative urodynamics, which was reduced to 18 percent in preferred practice. Eighty percent would operate a patient with a positive stress test without urodynamic SUI, whereas 21 percent would do this even with negative stress test. Only 9 percent would choose the type of sling based on UPP parameters (2% used MUCP, 42% used VLPP). Only 43 percent would interpret their ordered urodynamic results by themselves. 42 gynecologists (41%) were unable to interpret the curves of an urodynamic investigation, versus only 2 urologists (3%).[31]

According to current guidelines of EAU, clinicians carrying out urodynamics in patients with UI must ensure that the test replicates patient's symptoms. They should interpret results in context of the clinical problem and recordings should be checked for quality control. Physiological variability within the same individual should always be kept in mind [GR C]. Patients should be advised that the results may be useful in discussing treatment options, although there is limited evidence that it will alter the outcome of treatment for UI [GR C].[2]

Therefore urodynamics should not be routinely carried out when offering conservative treatment for UI [GR B][2] and for women with a clearly defined clinical diagnosis of pure stress UI [D].[1] It should be done only, if the findings may change the choice of surgical treatment; or prior to surgery for UI, if there are either symptoms of OAB, a history of previous surgery or a suspicion of voiding difficulty [D (GPP)][1] [GR C].[2]

Recently issued guidelines of American Urological Association (AUA) recommends to assess urethral function when making the diagnosis of urodynamic SUI (GR C), PVR when considering invasive therapy for SUI (expert opinion) and multichannel urodynamics when considering invasive, potentially morbid or irreversible treatments, in patients with UI (GR C).[14]

Stress testing with reduction of the prolapse should be done in women with high grade pelvic organ prolapse but without the symptom of SUI. Multichannel urodynamics with prolapse reduction may be used to assess for occult SUI and detrusor dysfunction in these women with associated LUTS (GR C). Repeat stress testing should be done after removing urethral catheter in patients suspected of having SUI with negative results during urodynamics (GR C). Pressure flow studies (PFS) should be considered in patients with UUI after bladder outlet procedures to evaluate for bladder outlet obstruction (expert opinion). Clinicians should counsel patients with UUI and MUI that the absence of DO on a single urodynamic study does not exclude it as a causative agent for their symptoms (clinical principle).[14]

Conclusion

Urodynamics are not routinely performed and guidelines on indications for urodynamics are not widely implemented, resulting in practice variation in work-up of women with UI. At present, the urodynamic outcomes hardly influence the choice of treatment. This indicates the necessity of conclusive evidence on whom to perform urodynamic investigation and how to combine different diagnostic modalities in a way to make evaluation less cumbersome, less invasive, less expensive, less time consuming and easy to access. Today's need is to perform more studies on current diagnostic modalities in order to create a more uniform work-up algorithm for UI.

References

1. NICE clinical guideline 40: The management of urinary incontinence in women, developed by the National Collaborating Centre for Women's and Children's Health, Issue date: October 2006.
2. Lucas MG, Bosch JLHR, Cruz FR, et al. EAU Guidelines on Urinary Incontinence, Issue date: Feb 2012.
3. Al Afraa T, Mahfouz W, Campeau L, et al. Review Article, Normal lower urinary tract assessment in women: I. Uroflowmetry and post-void residual, pad tests, and bladder diaries Int Urogynecol J. 2012;23:681-5.
4. Abrams P, Cardozo L, Fall M, et al. The standardisation of terminology of lower urinary tract function: report from the Standardisation Sub-committee of the International Continence Society. Neurourol Urodyn. 2002;21:167-78.
5. Sutherst J, Brown M, Shawer M. Assessing the severity of urinary incontinence in women by weighing perineal pads. Lancet. 1981;1:1128-30.
6. Moore EE, Jackson SL, Boyko EJ, et al. Urinary incontinence and urinary tract infection: temporal relationships in postmenopausal women. Obstet Gynecol. 2008:111 (2 Pt 1):317-23.

7. Ouslander JG, Schapira M, Schnelle JF, et al. Does eradicating bacteriuria affect the severity of chronic urinary incontinence in nursing home residents? Ann Intern Med. 1995;122(10):749-54.
8. Goode PS, Locher JL, Bryant RL, et al. Measurement of postvoid residual urine with portable transabdominal bladder ultrasound scanner and urethral catheterization. Int Urogynecol J Pelvic Floor Dysfunct. 2000; 11(5):296-300.
9. Ouslander JG, Simmons S, Tuico E, et al. Use of a portable ultrasound device to measure post-void residual volume among incontinent nursing home residents. J Am Geriatr Soc. 1994;42(11):1189-92.
10. Nygaard IE. Postvoid residual volume cannot be accurately estimated by bimanual examination. Int Urogynecol J Pelvic Floor Dysfunct. 1996; 7(2):74-6.
11. Griffiths DJ, Harrison G, Moore K, et al. Variability of post-void residual urine volume in the elderly. Urol Res. 1996;24(1):23-6.
12. Stoller ML, Millard RJ. The accuracy of a catheterized residual urine. J Urol. 1989;141(1):15-6.
13. Marks LS, Dorey FJ, Macairan ML, et al. Three-dimensional ultrasound device for rapid determination of bladder volume. Urology. 1997; 50(3):341-8.
14. Winters JC, Dmochowski RR, Goldman HB, Adult Urodynamics: American Urological Association (AUA) Guideline. Issue date: April 2012.
15. Saaby M L, Lose G. Repeatability of post-void residual urine ≥ 100 ml in urogynaecologic patients. Int Urogynecol J. 2012;23:207-20.
16. Woodfield CA, Krishnamoorthy S, Hampton BS, et al. Imaging pelvic floor disorders: trend toward comprehensive MRI. Am J Roentgenol. 2010;194(6):1640-9.
17. Morgan DM, Umek W, Guire K, et al. Urethral sphincter morphology and function with and without stress incontinence. J Urol. 2009;182(1):203-9.
18. Lewicky-Gaupp C, Blaivas J, Clark A, et al. "The cough game": are there characteristic urethrovesical movement patterns associated with stress incontinence? Int Urogynecol J Pelvic Floor Dysfunct. 2009;20(2):171-5.
19. Shek KL, Dietz HP, Kirby A. The effect of childbirth on urethral mobility: a prospective observational study. J Urol. 2010;184(2):629-34.
20. Shek KL, Chantarasorn V, Dietz HP. The urethral motion profile before and after suburethral sling placement. J Urol. 2010;183(4):1450-4.
21. Chantarasorn V, Shek KL, Dietz HP. Sonographic appearance of transobturator slings: implications for function and dysfunction. Int Urogynecol J. 2011;22(4):493-8.
22. Wein AJ, English WS, Whitemore KE. Office urodynamics. Urol Clin North Am. 1988;15:609.
23. Boone TB, Kim YH. Uroflowmetry. In: Nitti VW (Ed). Practical Urodynamics. Philadelphia: WB Saunders; 1998.pp.28-51.

24. Mahfouz W, Al Afraa T, Campeau L, et al. Normal urodynamic parameters in women Part II—invasive urodynamics. Int Urogynecol J. 2012;23:269-77.
25. Digesu GA, Khullar V, Cardozo L, Salvatore S. Overactive bladder symptoms: do we need urodynamics? Neurourol Urodyn. 2003; 22:105-8.
26. Price DM, Noblett K. Comparison of the cough stress test and 24-h pad test in the assessment of stress urinary incontinence. Int Urogynecol J. 2012;23:429-33.
27. Gamble TL, Botros SM, Beaumont JL, et al. Predictors of persistent detrusor overactivity after transvaginal sling procedures. Am J Obstet Gynecol. 2008;199(6):e691-7.
28. Smith AL, Jaffe WI, Wang M, et al. Detrusor overactivity leak point pressure in women with urgency incontinence. Int Urogynecol J. 2012; 23(4):443-6
29. Dietz HP, Shek KL. Levator function and voluntary augmentation of maximum urethral closure pressure. Int Urogynecol J. 2012; 23(8):1035-40.
30. Kapoor DS, Housami F, White P, et al. Maximum urethral closure pressure in women: normative data and evaluation as a diagnostic test. Int Urogynecol J. (2012) [Epub ahead of print].
31. Van Leijsen SA, Kluivers KB, Mol BW, et al. The value of preoperative urodynamics according to gynecologists and urologists with special interest in stress urinary incontinence. Int Urogynecol J. 2012;23 (4):423-8.

CHAPTER 5

Imaging in Urinary Incontinence

Sandeep Patil, Nishita Parekh, Prakash Trivedi

The term "imaging" is defined as the process of forming images on a computer screen, trying to reproduce an exact picture of a selected part of the body. Imaging modalities hold a crucial role in the diagnosis and management of several diseases, providing evidence regarding disease severity, indications for treatment and prognostic values. Moreover, they might be successfully used either to monitor patient conditions over time or to assess treatment outcomes during the follow-up as well as for research purposes. Imaging studies using ultrasound, plain X-ray, magnetic resonance imaging (MRI), computerized tomography (CT), isotopes and the most recent, virtual reality, have been proposed as tools to increase knowledge of the anatomy and physiology of normal lower urinary tract and the physiopathology of urinary incontinence and lower urinary tract dysfunction but till date, none has risen to the status of essential diagnostic procedure in the initial evaluation of uncomplicated urinary incontinence.

Urinary incontinence is "the compliant of any involuntary leakage of urine."[1] This simple definition hides an intrinsic complexity due to its multifactorial and still not completely clear etiology. In the initial evaluation of this condition, in the absence of coexisting other lower urinary tract dysfunctions and/or pelvic pathology, only the following tests are highly recommended.[2]

- History and general assessment
- Physical examination
- Urinalysis
- Symptoms quantification
- Quality of life assessment
- Assessment of the desire for treatment
- Estimation of postvoid residual (PVR) urine

Beyond these, further investigations are indicated only in selected patients.[3]

The assessment of the upper urinary tract using ultrasound, intravenous urography, CT, MRI and isotope scanning is not needed in the evaluation of uncomplicated stress, urge or mixed urinary incontinence. These studies aim at increasing the diagnostic requirements for invasive and specialized therapies and become an important part of the diagnostic evaluation in cases of neurogenic urinary incontinence or when any of the following conditions is suspected or diagnosed:[3]

- Dysfunctional voiding with significant PVR
- Coexisting loin/kidney pain
- Untreated severe pelvic organ prolapse (POP)
- Urodynamic studies showing a raised intravesical pressure on bladder filling.

Imaging techniques concerning the lower urinary tract, such as voiding cystourethrography (VCUG), videourodynamics, CT and MRI, may be indicated either when the upper urinary tract imaging studies are abnormal, or in cases of suspected pelvic floor dysfunction, particular systemic and/or pelvic diseases, previous failed surgery, recurrent posterior vaginal wall prolapse or to better assess urethra mobility. Voiding cystourethrography is useful for visualizing position and morphology of bladder, urethra and pelvic floor in female patients with urinary incontinence, but its real role in evaluating this condition is not yet established (although recent preliminary evidence highlighted a possible clinical utility of urethral angle and cystocele height measurement in the management of this kind of patient). VCUG is not able to discriminate between stress urinary incontinence and continent status, distinguish postoperative failures from success or disclose a correlation between the degree of stress urinary incontinence and the type or grade of suspension defects. For these reasons, this radiological procedure cannot be recommended for diagnosing and classifying urinary incontinence. Therefore, it is not indicated in primary uncomplicated stress, urge or mixed female urinary incontinence, but it may be considered as a reasonable option in the preoperative evaluation of complicated and/or recurrent female urinary incontinence and POP, in evident or suspected neurogenic urinary incontinence. Videourodynamics, using either ultrasound or X-ray imaging modalities, are an optional test eventually indicated in complicated or recurrent incontinence in children and neurologic patients. When it cannot be used, VCUG should be used as a separate test, although alone gives less information than videourodynamics, being unable to provide radiographs representative of functional states at appropriate moments.[3]

Ultrasound is frequently used for assessing female urinary incontinence and prolapse, and in skilled hands, it may provide useful functional and morphological information about the pelvic organs.

Ultrasound imaging, particularly using translabial or transperineal ultrasound access, will soon become a standard noninvasive diagnostic method in the evaluation of urogynecological dysfunction (**Figures 5.1A and B**).[4] A better assessment of levator ani activity and prolapse, and the use of translabial color Doppler to document urine leakage both are contributing factors in the improvement process of ultrasound in this field, enhancing its clinical usefulness. Moreover, the wide availability of suitable equipment, the ease of use, and the absence of adverse effects make this technique the most convenient imaging method currently available. By creating a coordinates system (x-axis as the central line of the pubis symphysis; y-axis perpendicular to the x-axis at the inferoposterior margin of the pubis symphysis; Dx as the distance between the y-axis and the bladder neck; Dy as the distance between the x-axis and the bladder neck; pubourethral (angle formed intersecting the x-axis with the urethra axis); urethrovesical (angle formed intersecting the urethra axis with the line tangential to the posterior bladder profile); and other rotation angles and distances proposed to improve the knowledge in this field) to quantify pelvic organ position and inclination angles between bladder, urethra and pubic bone, an ultrasonographic definition of the position and mobility of pelvic organs is possible, both at rest and on coughing or valsalva maneuver, better assessing female patients with urinary incontinence and prolapse before and after treatment (**Figures 5.2A and B**).

Ultrasound has become the imaging method of choice to identify the position of suburethral slings and other echogenic implants.

Ultrasound imaging for bladder neck descent, funneling and urine leakage seems to correlate well with radiological findings on fluoroscopy and cystourethrography. Moreover, a good correlation has been found between the assessment of maximal pelvic organ descent by translabial ultrasound and the International Continence Society Pelvic Organ Prolapse Quantification (ICS POP-Q) assessment. Pelvic floor ultrasound can be used to assess levator function and provide visual biofeedback for teaching pelvic floor muscle exercises. Three-dimensional (3D) ultrasound is an investigational tool that is able to rebuild structures in the axial plane such as paraurethral/paravaginal supports and the levator ani. Despite all these promising results, ultrasound is not currently recommended in the initial evaluation of patients with urinary incontinence and/or POP. Nevertheless, it represents a good optional test to assess patients with complex or recurrent urinary incontinence with or without POP. A better standardization of ultrasound imaging in incontinence, and knowledge of the relationship of ultrasound imaging to bladder neck and treatment outcome are suggested research areas to make this promising technique a diagnostic reality.[5]

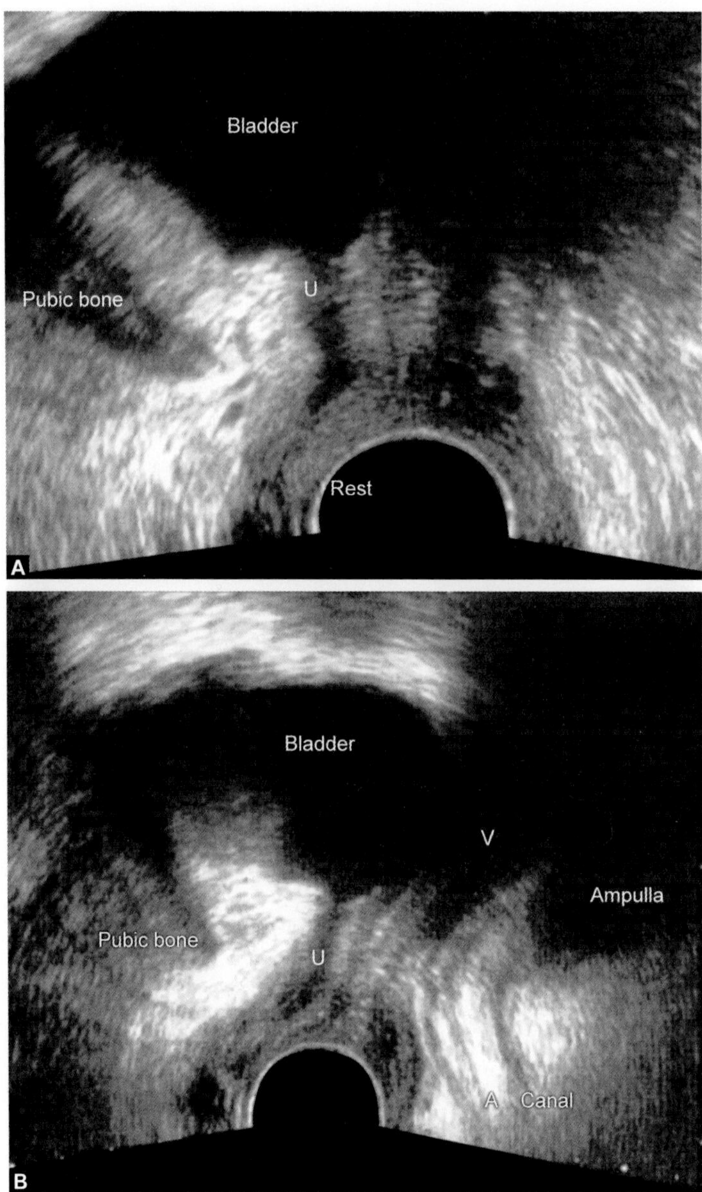

Figures 5.1A and B: Transperineal ultrasound imaging of bladder

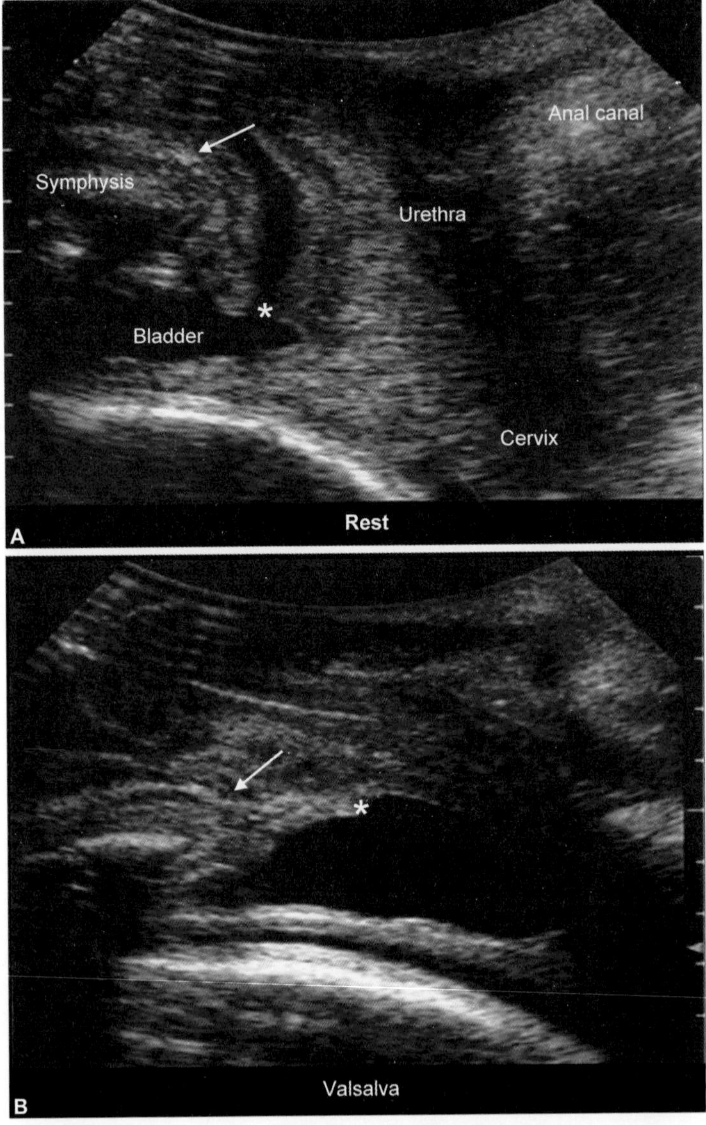

Figures 5.2A and B: Ultrasound comparative imaging of bladder neck

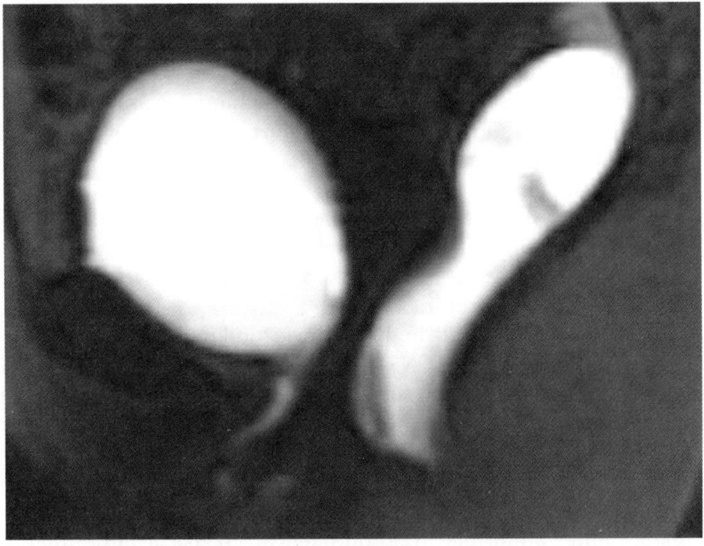

Figure 5.3: MRI visualization of bladder and urethral anatomy

Recently, CT has provided important information on the effect of straining on the posterior component of the levator ani, but the soft tissue details obtained by MRI are better. Therefore, CT as a research imaging method in pelvic floor studies has been abandoned.

MRI is an excellent, reproducible but expensive tool for assessing the female pelvis, including normal anatomy, pelvic floor relaxation and pelvic organ prolapse (**Figure 5.3**).

Dynamic MRI is helpful in evaluating persistent complaints after surgery for POP, and may be used to detect more defects than a physical examination or other imaging procedures. It may be useful in assessing stress urinary incontinence before and after surgery, reliably detecting possible associated anatomical changes. MRI should be considered when surgery has failed, in cases of severe POP, and to distinguish stress urinary incontinence due to bladder neck malposition from secondary to intrinsic sphincter damage. Three-dimensional MRI is able to easily visualize the overall pelvic structures, evaluating any pelvic floor weakness. MRI with endoluminal coil may reveal significant morphological changes in the supporting structures and the urethra in patients with stress urinary incontinence. Despite all these interesting and encouraging results, MRI is not yet indicated in the evaluation of patients with uncomplicated primary urinary incontinence or POP. MRI should still be considered an investigational imaging technique in the assessment of female urinary incontinence and pelvic floor dysfunction. It represents an excellent tool to better evaluate the following research standpoints:

- Anatomic changes involved in urinary incontinence and POP
- Effects of aging in support structures of the pelvis and their association with urinary incontinence and/or POP development
- Effects of surgery on pelvic anatomic changes and clinical outcomes
- Influence of pre- and postmenopausal hormonal environment on the pelvic support and urethra
- Structural relationship between spongy tissue and fibromuscular envelope of female urethra
- To better assess their role in the intrinsic function of the urethra.

Central nervous system (CNS) imaging covers a particular interest in research and in patients with suspected neurogenic lower urinary tract dysfunction, with or without abnormalities on neurological physical examination.

Lumbosacral X-rays should be indicated in children with suspected congenital neurogenic incontinence with or without gluteosacral stigmata and abnormal neurourological physical examination. Moreover, in all patients with suspected neurological disease, even with normal lumbosacral X-rays, a myelography or a CNS CT and/or MRI should be always considered. CNS CT, MRI, positron emission tomography (PET), and single-photon emission CT are all available tools useful in the diagnosis of a wide range of CNS diseases responsible for possible neurogenic lower urinary tract dysfunction, even in the absence of other obvious neurological symptoms. PET studies provide interesting information regarding specific brain regions involved in human micturition control. All these neuroimaging techniques should be considered only when a nervous system disorder is suspected on the basis of clinical and/or neurophysiological test findings.

Almost all the above-mentioned considerations, indications and recommendations regarding the different imaging modalities in the diagnosis and management of urinary incontinence are based on expert opinion or good quality retrospective "case-control studies" and good quality 'case series' (level of evidence four and three, respectively, and grade of recommendation C, according to the standard levels of evidence and grade of recommendations proposed by the Oxford Centre for Evidence Based Medicine and endorsed by the International Consultation on Urological Diseases).

Use of different imaging modalities often depends on availability, expertize and local management policies, instead of universally accepted guidelines.

Constant development, knowledge on functional and dysfunctional mechanisms will certainly improve, resulting in enhancement of the ability to take as much information as possible from the newest and future imaging techniques, finally obtaining more suitable reading keys.

References

1. Abrams PA, Cardozo L, Fall M, et al. The Standardization of terminology of lower urinary tract function: report from the standardization sub-committee of the International Continence Society, Neurourol. Urodyn. 2002;21:167-78.
2. Abrams P, Andersson KE, Brubaker L, et al. Recommendations of the International Scientific Committee. In: Abrams P, Cardozo L, Khoury S, Wein A (Eds), edition 2005, Incontinence 3rd International Consultation on Incontinence, 2004: pp.1589-629.
3. Tubaro A, Artibani W, Bertram C, Delancey JD, Dietz HP, Khullar V, Zimmer P, Umek U. Imaging and other Investigations. In: Abrams P, Cardozo L, Khoury S, Wein A (Eds), 2005, Incontinence 3rd International Consultation on Incontinence, 2004;13:707-97.
4. Vittorio Luigi Piloni, Liana Spazzafumo. Sonography of the female pelvic floor. Pelviperineology. 2007;26:59-65.
5. Hans Peter Dietz, et al. Pelvic floor ultrasound: a review. American Journal of Obsterics and Gynecology. 2010;202(4):321-34.

CHAPTER

6

Medical Management of Urinary Incontinence

Anita Patel

By definition, urinary incontinence (UI) is the demonstrable involuntary urinary loss that is socially and/or hygienically unacceptable to the patient or her caregivers. The International Continence Society (ICS) defines overactive bladder (OAB) as a complex of symptoms characterized by urgency, with or without urge incontinence, usually with frequency and nocturia, if there is no proven infection or other obvious pathology.[1] Worldwide, several studies report prevalence of urinary incontinence in the range 25 to 45 percent.[1] Stress urinary incontinence (SUI) is estimated to be the most prevalent type of UI, accounting for around 41 percent of cases; urge urinary incontinence (UUI) accounts for around 16 percent and mixed UI for around 34 percent of the total cases of incontinence.[2] SUI is more common in the younger age group and UUI is more common in the elderly. In 2006, the EPIC study reported the overall prevalence of storage urinary symptoms in 4 European countries and in Canada at 11.8 percent.[3] The National Overactive Bladder Evaluation (NOBLE) study in USA (2003) further clarified the prevalence of OAB in USA: the estimated prevalence is similar among men and women, 16 percent and 16.9 percent, respectively. In women, the prevalence of OAB with incontinence (OAB wet) ranges from 2 percent (aged 18–24 years) to 19 percent (aged 65–74 years), increasing markedly after age 44 years.[4]

As incontinence is not conventionally regarded as serious and in particular, as nobody dies from it, it used to be a low priority area till recently. However, better diagnostic modalities, better understanding of pathophysiology and availability of newer drugs have made a huge impact on improving the quality of life of these patients. The number of specialists interested in treating this condition is progressively increasing. As every patient with voiding dysfunction may or may not have incontinence, a better terminology coined by ICS is female lower urinary tract symptoms, also referred to as FLUTS. FLUTS includes both storage (frequency, urgency +/- incontinence) and voiding (slow flow, straining, incomplete emptying) symptoms. Following chapter gives a brief outline of medical management of various FLUTS and of course, urinary incontinence.[1,5]

Types of Urinary Incontinence

As with all voiding dysfunctions, incontinence can be considered as a malfunction of the bladder, the bladder outlet or both. Boldly, urinary incontinence can be subdivided into:

- *Stress urinary incontinence (SUI):* This refers to involuntary loss of urine with increase in abdominal pressure without any rise in detrusor pressure. An incompetent bladder outlet is usually responsible for this.
- *Urge urinary incontinence (UUI):* This refers to loss of urine due to an involuntary detrusor contraction, accompanied by an urge to void. This is due to detrusor overactivity (previously called instability), which may be idiopathic or secondary to neurogenic or non-neurogenic causes.
- *Mixed incontinence:* Here both SUI and UUI coexist in the same patient. However often one of them produces more bothersome symptoms.
- *Other types of incontinence:* These are, overflow incontinence and non-anatomic incontinence (leakage through a fistulous communication). Both these are relatively rare.

Physiology of Continence

In a woman, several factors help in maintaining continence. In the given list, the highlighted ones are where there is scope for medical or pharmacological manipulations.

- Resting tone of bladder neck and external urethral sphincter
- Anatomical intra-abdominal position of bladder neck and proximal urethra
- Hammock like support offered by the pelvic floor
- Intrinsic mucosal seal of the urethra, related to hormonal status
- A stable, and compliant urinary bladder
- Intact neurourological axis.

Disturbance in any of these factors can influence continence adversely. Thus aging, repeated deliveries, pelvic organ prolapse, systemic diseases such as diabetes, neurological disorders, can all produce incontinence. As the etiology is multifactorial, more than one factor is at play in any given patient. This can also explain why the same abnormality does not make every sufferer incontinent!

List of drugs with site of action

External sphincter: *Duloxetine (contraction), botulinum toxin (relaxation)*
Bladder neck: *Duloxetine, imipramin (contraction), alpha-blockers (relaxation)*
Detrusor muscle: *Antimuscarinics. (Tolterodine, solifenacin) botulinum toxin, smooth muscle relaxants (Oxybutinine, flavoxate)*

Physiological Basis of Pharmacological Intervention in Urinary Incontinence

During normal urination or voiding, the first event is permission by the cerebral hemispheres, leading to external sphincter relaxation (under somatic S2, 3, 4 control), followed by detrusor contraction (parasympathetic stimulation), followed by opening of the bladder neck (sympathetic relaxation), leading to urination. Thus unless there is higher center permission, urination cannot happen. Similarly, urinary storage happens when there is stimulation of sympathetic system (alpha-receptors closing the bladder neck, beta-receptors relaxing the detrusor); and inhibition of parasympathetic system.

Pharmacological agents can alter/improve the function of external sphincter, bladder neck and detrusor muscle.

External urethral sphincter is mainly composed of somatic muscles, which are directly under the control of pudendal nerves. Thus drugs acting either directly on the sphincter or at the neuromuscular junction or the sacral spinal center can be useful in altering its function. Imipramine and duloxetine improve the muscle contraction power, thus improving the continence. Detrusor muscle is mainly under the influence of parasympathetic autonomic system. The receptors are muscarinic type with 5 subtypes present (M1, M2, M3, M4, M5). The most prevalent receptors are M2 with most detrusor selective being M3. Stimulation of these receptors leads to detrusor contraction which in turn leads to urination provided there is permission from the higher centers. Involuntary detrusor contractions lead to urge incontinence. The drugs available in this category to block the muscarinic receptors and in turn to control the overactive detrusor contractions are pro-banthine, oxybutynin, tolterodine, solifenacin, darifenacin, trospium chloride. Beta sympathetic stimulants can be used for detrusor relaxation but in practice, alpha blockers with a weak beta action are used. Intradetrusor injection of Botulinum Toxin is useful in controlling detrusor over activity with a span of action lasting from 4 to 18 months. Rarely, there may be detrusor atonia due to myogenic failure, producing retention of urine. This may present as over flow incontinence. However cholinergic agents are not very useful in this situation due to unfavorable side effects.

Bladder neck mainly consists of smooth muscles which are under control of sympathetic nervous system. The receptor involved are alpha-adrenergic and these produce contraction of bladder neck, thus helping in staying continent at rest. A weakness of these muscles can produce incontinence and excessive contraction of these can produce slow flow and even retention. Thus both sympathomimetic and sympathetic receptor blocking agents help in voiding dysfunction as explained here. The drugs in this group are alpha-stimulants (Duloxetine, imipramine) and alpha-blockers (Prazosin, terazosin, doxazosin, alfuzosin, tamsulosin, and silodosin).

Estrogens may affect continence by increasing urethral resistance, raising the sensory threshold of bladder, increasing alpha-adrenoceptor sensitivity and ensuring a well-vascularized urethral mucosa as well as vaginal tissues.

Before starting medication for incontinence, one must understand that the key to successful management of any incontinence lies in correct diagnosis. Thus there are no shortcuts to correct history taking, detailed clinical examination followed by relevant investigations including a voiding diary, relevant urine and blood tests, bladder sonography and detailed urodynamic study with or without a video in appropriate situation. Once the diagnosis is confirmed, even prior to starting medication, certain conservative measures must be offered to all the patients ***(Figure 6.1)****. These include dietary and lifestyle changed, change in fluid drinking habits, weight loss measures, pelvic floor muscle training and biofeedback.*

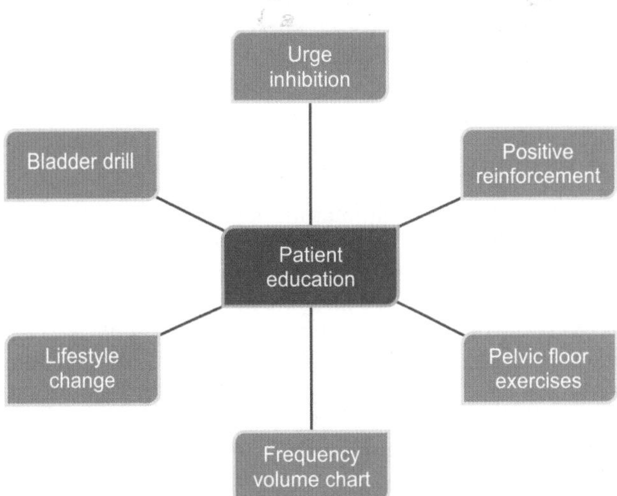

Figure 6.1: An integrated approach to conservative management of SUI as well as UUI, in addition to appropriate medication depending upon the cause

Medical Management

After appropriate evaluation, lifestyle modification and fluid intake advice must be given to all patients. Pelvic floor muscle exercises must be taught to all patients regardless of the type of incontinence, excluding over flow incontinence. There is adequate evidence in the literature supporting the use of all conservative measures in any form of incontinence, with Grade 1 B recommendation for the same in the EAU Guidelines 2012.[6] Patients in menopausal age group may be considered for local or systemic HRT. Adequate sugar control is absolutely essential in diabetics with urinary incontinence. Any urinary infection must be treated with appropriate antibiotics.

Estrogens and FLUTS

Female lower urinary tract shares a common embryological origin with the genital tract arising from the urogenital sinus. There are estrogen receptors found in the bladder, urethra, and pelvic floor in addition to the genital tract. Menopause and its associated estrogen deficiency are known to produce lower urinary tract symptoms (LUTS) in women starting anytime from 10 years before the menopause to years after menopause.[7] L Cardozo et al in a review article; looked at several RCTs to assess the effect of estrogen on symptoms of OAB in postmenopausal women.[8] The outcomes looked at were diurnal frequency, nocturnal frequency, incontinence episodes, urgency, first sensation to void, and bladder capacity. They concluded that all the aspects were improved by systemic or local HRT. However, interestingly estrogens are not very useful in the management of stress urinary incontinence. In fact there is evidence to prove that estrogens can actually worsen SUI![9]

Antimuscarinic Agents

Most of the neurohumoral stimulus for physiologic bladder contraction is from acetylcholine induced stimulation of postganglionic parasympathetic muscarinic cholinergic receptor sites on bladder smooth muscles. Atropine and atropine like agents inhibit normal and involuntary (overactive) bladder contractions of any etiology. Usually the volume to the first contraction increases, amplitude of the contraction decreases, and the total bladder capacity increases. This increases the warning time before a potential leak may start. Antimuscarinic agents also decrease the filling and storage symptomatology, unrelated to the occurrence of overactive detrusor contraction. Outlet resistance is unaffected by these agents.

The potential side effects of all antimuscarinic agents include inhibition of salivation, inhibition of ciliary and iris smooth muscle, tachycardia, drowsiness, cognitive dysfunction especially in the elderly, and inhibition of gut motility, often producing constipation. In general, these agents are contraindicated in patients with narrow angle glaucoma, and should be used with caution in those with significant bladder outlet obstruction.

- *Atropine sulfate:* This agent is rarely used to treat bladder overactivity due to its adverse systemic side effects.
- *Propantheline bromide:* One of the oldest known antimuscarinic agent used in urinary incontinence, it is now regarded as historic, mainly due to its poor side effect profile and availability of better drugs.
- *Tolterodine tartrate:* This agent was specifically developed for bladder, with some bladder selectivity. The usual adult dose is 2 mg twice a day. Newer extended release preparations make once a day dose feasible with a 2 mg and 4 mg option, with lesser incidence of side effects with equal efficacy. Tolterodine (2 mg or 4 mg extended release), when compared with placebo and 7.5 to 15 mg immediate release as well as extended release oxybutinin, was found to be superior in its efficacy (placebo), and side effect profile (oxybutinin).[10]
- *Trospium chloride:* This is a quaternary ammonium compound with nonreceptor selective antimuscarinic anticholinergic activity. As it does not cross the blood-brain barrier, it is safe in elderly population. The drug is now available in India as a 20 mg immediate release (12 hourly dosages) or 60 mg sustained release preparation (24 hourly dosages). The side effect profile is comparable to that of tolterodine and oxybutinin. Dmochowski et al in a placebo-controlled trial of 564 patients, found trospium to be effective in improving all symptoms of OAB.[11]
- *Solifenacin:* Solifenacin is one of the newer uroselective antimuscarinic agent, now available in the Indian market. Given in the dose of 5 to 10 mg once a day, it has comparable efficacy with tolterodine with a better side effect profile. The STAR study compared 4 mg extended release tolterodine with 5 mg of solifenacin and found better efficacy as well as tolerability.[12] Haab et al in a 12 weeks placebo-controlled double blind trial of solifenacin, in 1802 patients showed excellent long-term tolerability as well as acceptable side effect profile.[13]
- *Darifenacin:* This is a highly selective M3 receptor antagonist, thus believed to be the most specific agent available so far in the drug treatment of overactive bladder. It does not cross blood-brain barrier because of its large molecule size. Thus, like trospium, it is safer in elderly population. Foote et al in a prospective double blind randomized placebo-controlled study showed its efficacy as well as acceptable side effect profile with no CNS or cardiac side effects.[14]

The recommended daily dose is 7.5 or 15 mg once a day.

An ideal antimuscarinic agent is the one with maximum efficacy, minimum side effects with once a day dosage and long-term safety. Unfortunately, none of the agents currently available in the market qualify for the same. In practice, one must consider safety of any medication first, before looking into its efficacy and other factors.

Anticholinergics (Antimuscarinics) with Mixed Actions

These agents have a direct antispasmodic action on smooth muscle at a site that is metabolically distal to cholinergic or other contractile receptor mechanism; most probably related to calcium channel blockade. However, their therapeutic effects occur mainly through the antimuscarinic effect.

- *Oxybutinin chloride:* This is a potent muscarinic receptor antagonist with some degree of selectivity for M1 and M3 receptors. In human tissues, it has a higher tissue affinity for the receptors in the salivary gland than those in the bladder. This agent is a well-absorbed, tertiary amine with extensive first pass liver metabolism. The active metabolite is thought to cause most of its adverse effects. Hence intravescical, transdermal as well as rectal preparations are available, which bypass the liver and reduce the metabolite mediated side effects significantly. The recommended daily adult dose is 2.5 to 5 mg 3 times a day. The main bothersome side effects range from dry mouth to constipation and cognitive impairment. Like tolterodine, once daily preparations are available as oxybutinin ER or XL (5 mg, 7.5 mg, 10 mg and 15 mg). These have an innovative osmotic drug delivery system to release the drug at a controlled rate over a 24-hour period; with fewer side effects. Various trials have shown superior efficacy profile and improved side effect profile of these preparations over the immediate release preparation.[10]
- *Flaoxate hydrochloride:* A historically popular agent in the treatment of detrusor overactivity, it acts mainly by a direct smooth muscle relaxing effect on the detrusor as well as by exerting a local anesthetic effect. The antimuscarinic effect in the therapeutic dose is minimum. However, with availability of better drugs, nowadays this agent is used relatively less frequently.

Tricyclic Antidepressants

These have central and peripheral anticholinergic effects at some sites, they prevent the reuptake of released norepinephrine and serotonin and they are sedatives. All of the above effects are relevant in the treatment of urinary incontinence. Imipramine is the only relevant drug from this group, suitable for treatment of both OAB and SUI.

Imipramine: Though not a very potent bladder antimuscarinic agent, it has strong direct smooth muscle relaxing effect on the detrusor, which is neither cholinergic, nor adrenergic. This is probably related to increased serotonin activity in the CNS. It also increases outlet resistance by directly acting on the external sphincter, making it suitable in SUI. The usual dose is 25 to 75 mg per day. The main side effects are anticholinergic; the uncommon side effects are cardiac toxicity, CNS effects, postural hypotension, weakness and fatigue. As elderly patients with incontinence may be on multiple cardiac, neurological drugs, a close consultation with the patient's physician is necessary. Long term use of these as primary treatment of urinary incontinence is not recommended.

Miscellaneous Agents

Drugs such as potassium channel openers, calcium antagonists, prostaglandin inhibitors, Beta-adrenergic agonists, etc. are in theory capable of modifying the detrusor activity and be effective in the management of OAB. However in practice, the required dose and associated side effect profile makes them unsuitable for clinical usage. Drugs to decrease sensory input such as capsaicin or hot red pepper extract are more useful in cases of interstitial cystitis. Drugs such as ephedrine, pseudoephedrine, and phenylpropanolamine can be used to increase outlet resistance in SUI; but due to serious concerns about hypertensive side effect of these agents, they are not recommended for treatment of urinary incontinence.

Serotonin-Noradrenalin Reuptake Inhibitor

Duloxetine: Duloxetine is a potent and balanced dual serotonin and norepinephrine reuptake inhibitor (SNRI) that enhances urethral rhabdosphincter activity and consequently the bladder capacity in a cat bladder model. Clinically, duloxetine 80 mg per day (40 mg twice daily) decreases the incontinence episode frequency (IEF) and improves incontinence-related quality of life (I-QoL) independent of baseline incontinence severity and also in patients awaiting surgery. The onset of action is within 1 to 2 weeks. Nausea is the most common treatment emergent adverse event. This is mostly experienced early after the start of duloxetine (usually within the first few days) and is usually mild or moderate and nonprogressive in severity. The majority of patients reporting nausea continue treatment with duloxetine and in most of these patients the nausea resolves within 1 to 4 weeks. The drug can also be started at 20 mg twice a day and slowly increased to the therapeutic dose. It is also available in a sustained release preparation of 60 mg SR.

Cochrane systematic review 2005 performed a meta-analysis of nine randomized trials, involving 3327 adults with predominantly SUI, randomized to receive duloxetine or placebo. It was revealed that duloxetine was significantly better than placebo in terms of improving patients' quality of and perception of improvement. Individual studies demonstrated a significant reduction in the incontinence episode frequency (IEF) by approximately 50 percent during treatment with duloxetine. With regard to objective cure, however, meta-analysis of stress pad test and 24 hours pad weight change failed to demonstrate a benefit for duloxetine over placebo though data were relatively few. They concluded that the available evidence suggests that duloxetine treatment can significantly improve the quality of life of patients with stress urinary incontinence, but it is unclear whether or not benefits are sustainable. Adverse effects are common but not serious. Thirty percent patients reported side effects, mainly nausea and sedative effects and about 12 percent stopped treatment as a consequence. Currently, duloxetine is approved only for short-term treatment of SUI.[15]

Medication for Voiding FLUTS

As there are alpha-receptors mainly in the bladder neck, it seems logical to use these in rare cases where FLUTS are due to bladder neck obstruction, along with both storage and voiding symptoms. This is similar to its usage in male patients with prostatic hyperplasia with detrusor over activity. Amongst the available agents, terazosin (2 mg one or twice a day) and tamsulosin (0.4 mg or 0.8 mg) have been studied in this regard and have been found to be useful. The EAU guidelines make a grade "C" recommendation for their use in FLUTS, which means their usage is optional. As regards to their role in improving emptying, the clinically seen effects are at best modest. Though the newer agents are highly selective for alpha 1A and alpha 1D receptors, with minimal side effect profile, postural drop in blood pressure may still be seen in some cases. In general these drugs are tolerated very well.[16] However by lowering outlet resistance; all alpha blockers have the ability to worsen any urinary incontinence, especially SUI.[17]

Botulinum Toxin

Botulinum toxin is a neurotoxin, produced by *Clostridium botulinum*. It prevents the release of acetyl choline at the neuromuscular junction, thus preventing the subsequent muscle contraction. This agent has been increasingly used in cases of both neurogenic and non-neurogenic detrusor over activity as well as in cases of refractory OAB. The patients undergoing this treatment should be counseled about its potential side effect of retention of urine as well as the possible need for self- catheterization. The fact that it is a temporary treatment with reported benefit lasting from 3 to 15 months has to be emphasized, thus underlining the need for repeat injections. The dose varies from 100 to 300 units per sitting, injected cystoscopically at 10 to 30 sites in the detrusor, sparing the trigone. Mohanty et al showed the efficacy of botox injection in OAB in 39 cases with benefit lasting from 6 to 9 months.[18] Shahid Khan et al reported patient perceived outcome at 4 weeks after injecting 200 units of Botox and reported complete continence in >50 percent cases of refractory OAB.[19]

Management of Overflow Incontinence

This situation is often encountered in clinical practice in elderly frail women, often bed bound due to various other comorbidities. Common causes are mechanical issues such as external pressure due to a loaded rectum, urethral narrowing, an unrecognized pelvic organ prolapse and age-related detrusor dysfunction. Management initially involves inserting an indwelling catheter, especially if there is upper tract dilatation with infection and raised creatinine, etc. Once the patient stabilizes, the options are between continuing indwelling catheter either via urethral or suprapubic route and intermittent catheterization. The most practical option in an individual situation must be suggested. Medication rarely helps reversing the behavior of a chronically stretched detrusor but any mechanical cause (fecal impaction, third degree prolapse) must be corrected followed by a catheter free trial. Some patients with chronic retention may benefit by a temporary catheterization followed by catheter free trial. Some patients may need intermittent urethral dilatation if indeed there is proven urethral stenosis.

Standard Management of Storage LUTS

All patients must be advised regarding dietary and lifestyle changes, importance of weight loss, bio-feedback and PFME. In addition, anti-muscarinic should be started in clear cases of clinical diagnosis of OAB, with a follow-up visit after 4 weeks. Depending on their response and presence of any adverse effects, any change in the medication can be considered. Responders should be encouraged to continue all treatment aspects for 3 to 4 months, after which medication can be tapered and finally stopped. There would be cases requiring antimuscarinic medication on a long-term basis and safety of these is proven in such circumstances. Darifenacin and trospium are preferred in elderly patients. Patients resistant to the above management are labeled as resistant OAB. Management of resistant OAB involves looking into patient compliance, emphasizing the need for PFME and lifestyle modification, changing over to another antimuscarinic agent and finally considering invasive treatment options from botulinum toxin injection to surgical options such as augmentation cystoplasty.

Standard Management of Voiding LUTS

Patients with proven slow flow and significant residue should be first assessed to rule out mechanical causes of bladder outlet obstruction such as urethral stenosis and high grade pelvic organ prolapse producing a bladder neck kink (this being a more common clinical situation). Such patients clearly merit appropriate surgical intervention. Once mechanical problem is ruled out, patients can be started on alpha blockers. After a trial of medication for 4 weeks, patients can be reviewed with repeat flowmetry and residual urine evaluation. The responders should continue the medication and be on regular follow-up. The non-responders should be considered for surgical bladder neck incision after demonstrating a closed bladder neck on the voiding film of an MCU.

Management of Mixed Urinary Incontinence

In practice it is often seen that both urge and stress incontinence co-exist. The trick is in making the correct diagnosis. The treatment strategy is very simple, depending mainly on which symptoms predominate and bother the patients the most. After the standard lifestyle change, bladder drill and PFME, etc. usually antimuscarinics should be started as first line treatment. Topical and rarely systemic HRT may be used in selected postmenopausal patients. Depending on symptomatic response, further targeted therapy can be decided. This allows some time for the patient to start and continue both medication and PFME as a part of their routine. Those with true detrusor over activity will automatically report significant symptomatic improvement, thus further refining the role of surgery in appropriate cases of SUI.

Summary

Above text is a brief outline of medical management of various LUTS in female patients. All components including lifestyle change, weight reduction, fluid restriction, PFME and medication play a very important role as mentioned above. Any treatment strategy has to be individualized for each patient to achieve optimum treatment outcome. It is also equally important to identify those cases which clearly need surgical intervention, well on time. Such an approach would truly define ideal urogynecological management of these patients.

References

1. Abrams P, Cardozo L, Fall M, et al. The standardization of terminology of lower urinary tract function: report from the standardization sub-committee of the international continence society. Neurourol Urodyn. 2002;21:167-78.
2. National Collaborating Centre for Women's and Children's Health Urinary incontinence. Full national clinical guideline on the management of urinary incontinence in women. 2006, London: RCOG Press.
3. Irwin I, Milsom K, Reilly K, et al. Prevalence of overactive bladder syndrome: European results from the epic study. European Urology. 2006;5 (Suppl.): 115.
4. Stewart WF, Van Rooyen JB, Cundiff GW, Abrams P, Herzog AR, Corey R, et al. Prevalence and burden of overactive bladder in the United States. World J Urol. 2003;20:327-36.
5. Moller LA, Lose G, Jorgensen T. The prevalence and bothersomeness of lower urinary tract symptoms in women 40-60 years of age. Acta Obstet Gynecol Scand. 2000;79:298-305.
6. Lucas MG, et al. Guidelines on urinary incontinence. EAU guidelines 2012.
7. Dudley Robinson, Cardozo L. Hormonal Influences on Continence, Continence, 2009, II, Chapter 6, 65-83.
8. Cardozo L, Lose G, McClish D, Versi E. A systematic review of the effects of estrogens for symptoms suggestive of overactive bladder. Acta Obstet Gynecol Scand. 2004;83:892-7.
9. Moeher B, Hextall A, Jackson S. Estrogens for urinary incontinence in women, Cochrane review. In: Cochrane Library, Issue 3, Oxford: Update software.
10. Chapple CR, Khullar V, et al. The effects of antimuscarinic treatments in overactive bladder: an update of a systematic review and meta-analysis. Eur Urol. 2008;54:543-62.
11. Dmochowski RR, Sand PK, Zinner NR, Staskin DR. Trospium 60 mg once daily (QD) for overactive bladder syndrome: results from a placebo-controlled interventional study. Urol. 2008;71(3):449-54.
12. Chapple CR, Fianu-Jonsson A, Indig M, Khullar V, Rosa J, Scarpa RM, Mistry A, Wright DM, Bolodeoku J. STAR study group. Treatment

outcomes in the STAR study: a sub-analysis of Solifenacin 5 mg and Tolterodine ER 4 mg. Eur Urol. 2007;52(4):1195-203.
13. Haab F, Cardozo L, Chapple C, Ridder AM. Solifenacin Study Group. Long-term open-label Solifenacin treatment associated with persistence with therapy in patients with overactive bladder syndrome. Eur Urol. 2005;47(3):376-84.
14. Foote J, Glavind K, Kralidis G, Wyndaele JJ. Treatment of overactive bladder in the older patient: pooled analysis of three phase III studies of Darifenacin, an M3 selective receptor antagonist. European Urology. 2005;48(3):471-7.
15. Mariappan P, Ballantyne Z, N'Dow JM, Alhasso AA. Serotonin and noradrenaline reuptake inhibitors (SNRI) for stress urinary incontinence in adults. Cochrane Database Syst Rev. 2005;(3):CD004742.
16. Low BY, Liong ML, Yuen KH, et al. Terazosin therapy for patients with female lower urinary tract symptoms: A randomized, double-blind, placebo-controlled trial. J Urol. 2008;179:1461-9.
17. Dwyer PL, Teele JS. Prazosin: A neglected cause of genuine stress incontinence. Obstet Gynaecol. 1992;79:117-21.
18. Mohanty NK, Rajiba L Nayak, Mohd Alam, Arora RP. Role of botulinum toxin-A in management of refractory idiopathic detrusor overactive bladder: Single center experience. Indian Jour Urol. 2008;24(2):182-5.
19. Shahid Khan, Jalesh Panicker, Alexander Roosen, Gwen Gonzales, Sohier Elneil, Prokar Dasgupta, Clare J Fowler, Thomas M Kessler. Complete Continence after Botulinum Neurotoxin Type A Injections for Refractory Idiopathic Detrusor Over activity Incontinence: Patient-Reported Outcome at 4 Weeks. Eur Urol. 2010;57(5):735-920.

CHAPTER

7

Experience of Open Burch

Vivek Joshi

Though conservative management (pelvic floor muscle) may be useful in lower grades of stress urinary incontinence (SUI), surgery is the mainstay for treatment of SUI. In recent years, the treatment of women with SUI has undergone many changes as newer surgical techniques have been developed with the aim to offer good long-term results, reduced hospital stay and quicker return to normal activity.

Modified Burch Colposuspension

The prevalence of urinary incontinence varies from 10 to 40 percent but can be over 50 percent in elderly women. Multiple theories have been put-forth for explaining the pathophysiology of SUI and similar number of surgical procedures developed for its' treatment. However, Burch colposuspension procedure has withstood the test of time and has retained prominence in surgical armamentarium. In fact, it is considered a gold standard by most urogynecologist in the management of SUI, to which other surgical techniques can be compared.

Historical Aspect: To be Copied

Pathophysiology

Normal continence in women is a result of coordination of urinary bladder, urethra, pelvic muscles and surrounding connective tissue. The mechanisms for SUI are complex and not entirely understood. Although, SUI is either due to bladder neck hypermobility or intrinsic sphincter deficiency, most agree that some degrees of intrinsic sphincter deficiency (ISD) are present in all women with stress incontinence and the goal of incontinence surgery is to increase outlet obstruction achieved either by repositioning the bladder neck to its correct anatomical position (as in

Burch colposuspension) as to create a hammock against which urethra gets compressed during straining (as in pubovaginal or midurethral sling procedure like TVT or TOT) less invasive as compared to Burch colposuspension and give equally good success rates. However the erosion rates of the currently used polypropylene tapes are quite high, which can lead to pain, dyspareunia, vaginal discharge and urinary tract infections.

Preoperative Evaluation

Burch colposuspension gives optimum long-term results in properly selected cases.

Type 1 SUI when there is predominantly bladder neck hypermobility. This can be diagnosed by proper history, positive Bonney's test, transperineal ultrasound examination and in selected cases urodynamic evaluation to know the presence of associated detrusor instability and measure maximum urethral closure pressure and abdominal leak point pressure. Maximum urethral closure pressure <20 cm of water or abdominal leak point pressure <60 cm of water signify intrinsic sphincter deficiency as the predominant component responsible for SUI. In such situation, pubovaginal or midurethral sling procedures are preferred to Burch colposuspension.

If urodynamic studies are not available one can do Burch colposuspension under following circumstances: (a) No history suggestive of urge incontinence (b) Urine leaks from urethra in spurts with increase in abdominal pressure and leak stops as soon as patient stops coughing (c) Positive Bonney's test with good vaginal capacity and mobility (d) Transperineal USG confirms presence of hypermobile bladder neck.

Steps

- Exposure of retropubic space.
- Identification of pectineal ligament.
- Dissection of bladder medially off the vagina
- Placement of nonabsorbable suture through the vaginal at the bladder neck
- Suspending the vagina and fascia to the ipsilateral pectineal ligament.

Surgical Technique of Modified Burch Colposuspension

Modified lithotomy position is used with surgeon standing on the left side and second assistant on the right side. After thorough painting of abdomen, perineum and vagina wit 10 percent povidone iodine. Foley's catheter 16 Fr is inserted and the balloon inflated with 10 cc of distilled water to precisely know the position of bladder neck.

- Retropubic space is exposed using De Cherneys' incision.
- Pectineal ligament on both sides is cleared off the fat and loose areolar using blunt dissection with gauze. Pectineal ligament (Cooper's ligament) are strong thick fibrous bands running along the superior ramus of the pubic bone on either side. The lateral 1 to 2 cm of the ligament are utilized in this surgical technique (**Figure 7.1**).
- Index and middle finger of the left hand are in the vagina to elevate the anterior vaginal wall near the left vaginal fornix. Facilitated by the counter-pressure given by the vaginal fingers, the bladder base is dissected off the paravaginal fascia and the vagina at the level of bladder neck. The Foley balloon serves as a landmark for identification of bladder neck. In a primary procedure the dissection is effortless and once the bladder is dissected medially, the vagina with its covering fascia is easily identified by virtue of its white appearance and firm texture. All the vesical veins should be pushed medially along with the bladder muscle. In case bleeding occurs from one of such veins, homeostasis is achieved by under running these veins with chromic catgut 1.0. Use of diathermy is not advisable as it can provoke brisk hemorrhage from torn veins. If there has been a prior surgical attempt in the retropubic space the resultant fibrosis may make blunt dissection between the bladder and vagina difficult and in such situation sharp scissor dissection in the proper plane is necessary.

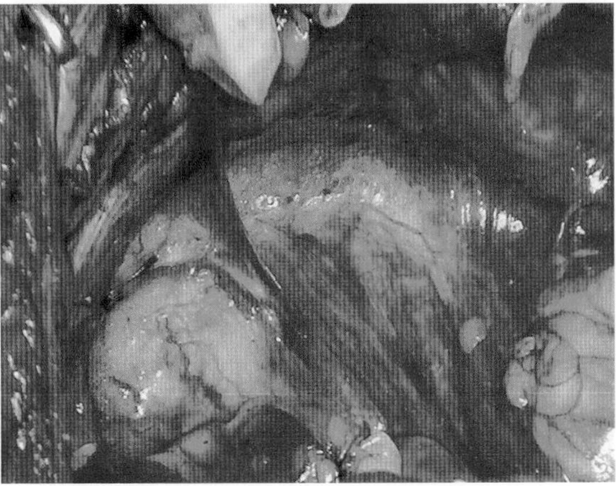

Figure 7.1: Pectineal ligament/Cooper's ligament

- Polypropylene number 1 sutures are now passed through the entire thickness of the vagina at the level of midpoint of Foley's balloon (**Figure 7.2**). A single mattress "figure-of-8" suture placed at the exact location is sufficient to give good long-term results. Even when the Prolene sutures include entire thickness of vaginal wall, epithelialization consistently occurs over such sutures so that they neither visible nor palpable in the postoperative period. The suture passed through the vagina is now tied first on the vagina itself to achieve hemostasis and minimize the risk of suture pulling through the vaginal tissue.
- The prolene suture passed through the vagina at the bladder neck is now passed through adequate portion of the most lateral ipsilateral pectineal ligaments.
- Using the same the same technique, a prolene no 1 suture is passed through the vagina on the right side of the bladder neck and then through the right pectineal ligament.
- Sutures on either side are now drawn taut so as to elevate the vagina and paravaginal fascia to the ipsilateral pectineal ligament and are firmly anchored here with 4 to 5 knots.
- Once the suspension sutures are tied one can clearly see the elevation of bladder neck (Foley balloon) to a high retropubic place and this guarantees good long-term cure rates.
- At completion of colposuspension the surgeon should be able to pass two fingers between the Foley balloon and the posterior side of pubic symphysis. The Foley balloon should move free in and out. Once this

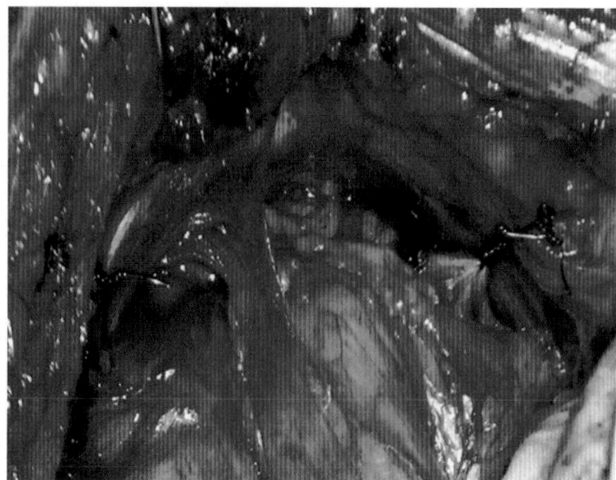

Figure 7.2: Polypropylene number 1 sutures passed through the entire thickness of the vagina at the level of midpoint of Foley's balloon

is confirmed one can be sure that there would not be any voiding difficulty.

Concomitant Surgical Procedure with Burch Colposuspension

In addition to this technique of Burch colposuspension other procedures like hysterectomy, Moschcowitz suture, uterine suspension and posterior colpoperineorrhaphy can be done when indicated. The sequence of various concomitant procedures should be:

- Abdominal hysterectomy/Uterine suspension
- Modified Burch colposuspension
- Moschcowitz or Halban's culdoplasty for enterocele
- Posterior colpoperineorrhaphy.

After doing Burch colposuspension following concomitant abdominal hysterectomy the vaginal vault should be carefully inspected for any bleeding points. Similarly enterocele should be taken care of since Burch colposuspension tends to exaggerate enterocele. However it is unnecessary to take Moschcowitz suture in all cases following Burch colposuspension. Rectocele repair if needed is done at the end to prevent contamination of the abdominal wound from perineum.

Operative Difficulties and their Management

- The key to successful outcome in Burch colposuspension is excellent exposure of the retropubic space. Though the procedure can be done either by a Pfannenstiel or midline incision the author feels that only a Cherney's incision gives best exposure to the space. There are two main advantages of optimum exposure.
  - Vesical veins can be easily under-run in case hemorrhage occurs. Good exposure use of suction and proper illumination of operative field (fiberoptic light source can be useful) make hemostasis easy. Pressure using sponges may decrease the hemorrhage. However proper identification and ligation of bleeding vessel is required for proper control of hemorrhage and prevent postoperative hematomas.
  - Good exposure facilitates precise placement of suspension sutures at the bladder neck which is needed for successful surgical outcome.
- Ideally, Burch colposuspension should be selected when the vaginal capacity and mobility is not restricted. However, if the preoperative judgment was incorrect, and if one finds that the vagina cannot be

elevated adequately up to the pectineal ligament a vagino-obturator shelf procedure can be performed by suturing the vagina to the obturator fascia instead of pectineal ligaments. The long-term results of the vagino-obturator shelf procedures are not as good as Burch colposuspension, since the obturator fascia is not as strong as the pectineal ligament.

- *Bladder laceration:* During colposuspension the possibility of bladder injury exists in two situations. The first is when bladder is being dissected medially off the vagina if one dissects in the wrong plane and uses too much force. This can especially happen because to fibrosis due to prior surgery I the retropubic space. Secondly, it is extremely important to differentiate between the strong white firm vagina and the pale yellow bladder, otherwise part of vesical wall can be included with the vagina in the prolene sutures, this suture should be cut first and then bladder should be further dissected medially. Once the vagina is identified, suture can be properly placed through the vagina and tied to pectineal ligament.

Outcome

The open Burch procedure has the best documentation of long-term success. Urodynamic testing confirms long-term success rates of 70 to 90 percent for women with mixed incontinence or those who have previous failed incontinence surgery. These findings were illustrated by a meta-analysis of seven studies with a follow-up 5 to 12 years that reported a cure rate of 90 percent for primary Burch colposuspension versus 82 percent for repeat surgery. Obesity, asthma age more than 65 years and estrogen deficiency are additional factors which lower the success rates.

Complications

- Postoperative voiding dysfunction and detrusor instability both appear to be related to excessive bladder neck elevation and urethral compression. The nerve damage associated with extensive dissection and placement of sutures caudal to bladder neck may result in funneling of the bladder neck causing *de novo* detrusor instability. The precise placement of suspension sutures at the bladder neck can prevent these complications. In my experience postoperative voiding difficulty are rare (2 cases). They occurred after Burch colposuspension which was done in patients who had undergone hysterectomy in past. If there is significant residual urine and with total inability to pass one month after surgery urethrolysis is necessary. In the procedure of urethrolysis releasing incisions are taken through the entire thickness of vagina on either side at lateral vaginal fornix. This releases the compression force on the urethra and voiding difficulty gets cured.

- *Postoperative enterocele:* The incidence varies from 3 to 17 percent. It is postulated that Burch colposuspension changes the axis of the posterior vaginal wall, exposing it to greater degree of intra-abdominal pressure. In women with deep pouch of Douglas, prophylactic culdoplasty sutures should be used.

Key Points

- Modified Burch colposuspension gives more than 90 percent long-term cure in properly selected women with SUI. (Predominantly bladder neck hypermobility, positive Bonney's test, good vaginal capacity and mobility).
- A single figure-of-eight suture exactly at the bladder neck incorporates entire thickness of vagina and suspending it to the most lateral part of ipsilateral part of pectineal ligament is necessary for good surgical outcome.
- If intraoperative hemorrhage occurs, bleeding vessels should be under run which is easy due to excellent exposure of retropubic space through Cherney's incision.
- Postoperative voiding difficulty may occur if suspension suture are placed caudal to bladder neck with urethra getting compressed against the pubic symphysis. In such situations urethrolysis is necessary for relieve obstruction.

Conventional Surgery and Biological Slings for Stress Urinary Incontinence

Yugali Warade, Sarika Dodwani, Prakash Trivedi

Introduction

Surgeons currently use a number of materials for constructing pubovaginal slings, with excellent outcomes. All types of stress urinary incontinence (SUI) may be corrected with pubovaginal sling surgery. Serious complications from sling surgery are uncommon. The choice of sling material and sling surgery is predominantly one of surgeon preference, the condition of host fascia/tissue, and previous surgery. The ideal sling material to use and the method of fixation are controversial.

Von Giordano is usually credited with performing the first pubovaginal sling operation in 1907, using a gracilis muscle graft around the urethra. In 1914, Frangenheim used rectus abdominis muscle and fascia for pubovaginal slings. In 1942, Aldridge, Millin, and Read corrected urinary incontinence using fascial slings. In 1965, Zoedler and Boeminghous first introduced synthetic slings. Historically, surgeons have used the rectus fascia pubovaginal sling for complex SUI after a failed anti-incontinence operation. In addition, surgeons performed this operation extensively for treatment of primary intrinsic sphincter deficiency (ISD).

Despite originating as an autologous procedure, many different types of materials have been used as sling substitutions, including various sources of autologous tissue, allograft tissue, xenograft tissue, and synthetic material. Almost all these substitutions have been made in an attempt to limit patient morbidity by alleviating the additional morbidity created by the harvesting of the sling material.

Nevertheless, the most popular pubovaginal sling still uses autologous rectus abdominis fascia. Regardless of the material used, the pubovaginal sling is meant to be placed at the junction of the proximal urethra and bladder neck for purposes of supporting the urethra, as well as augmenting intraurethral pressure and deficient proximal sphincteric function.

Mechanism of action

Direct compressive force on the urethra/bladder outlet or by re-establishing a reinforcing platform or hammock against which the urethra is compressed during transmission of increased abdominal pressure.

Indications

- *Intrinsic sphincter deficiency*
- *Urethral hypermobility*
- *Recurrent SUI after a synthetic sling surgery/complication*
- *Postradiation*
- *Concurrent or prior urethrovaginal fistula or diverticulum repair*
- *Adjunct for urethral and bladder reconstruction*

Mechanism of Action

The anterior distal wall of the urethra is attached to the pubic bone by the pubourethral ligaments **(Figure 8.1)**. These ligaments consist of extension of the perineal membrane and the caudal and ventral—most portion of the ATFP. The ligaments may limit movement of the anterior wall of the urethra during increases in intra-abdominal pressure but probably exert a lesser degree of support to the posterior wall.

Continence is achieved either by providing a direct compressive force on the urethra/bladder outlet or by re-establishing a reinforcing platform or hammock against which the urethra is compressed during transmission

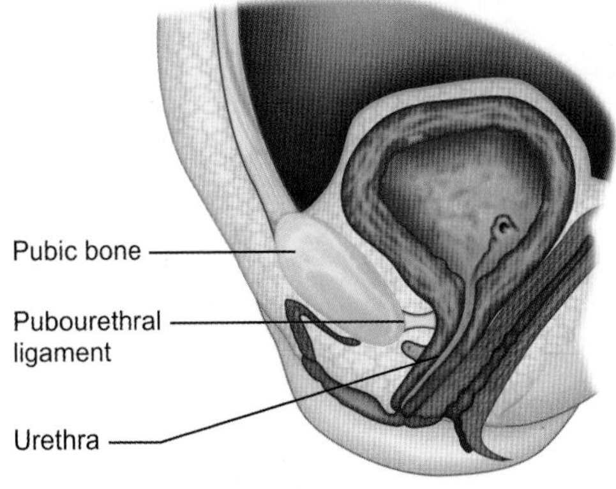

Figure 8.1: The pubourethral ligaments suspend the female urethra under the pubic arch

of increased abdominal pressure. The sling is suspended with free sutures on each end that either, is attached directly to the abdominal wall musculature or more commonly are tied to each other on the anterior surface of the abdominal wall **(Figure 8.2)**. The long-term success of the procedure relies not on the integrity of the suspensory sutures, but rather on the healing and fibrotic process involving the sling, which occurs primarily where the sling passes through the endopelvic fascia.

Indications

The pubovaginal sling is a treatment option for stress urinary incontinence (SUI). Although pioneered as a surgical option for intrinsic sphincter deficiency, the indications have been broadened to encompass all types of SUI. Because of its reliable results and durable outcomes, it is considered to be one of the main standards of treatment of SUI and has been used extensively as a primary therapy of SUI both for intrinsic sphincter deficiency and for urethral hypermobility, as a salvage procedure for recurrent SUI, as an adjunct for urethral and bladder reconstruction, and even as a way to "close" the urethra functionally to abandon urethral access to the bladder altogether.

In our opinion, other indications are in patients with SUI who decline to have a synthetic material implanted because of concerns related to the long-term presence of synthetic mesh. Also, women who have recurrent

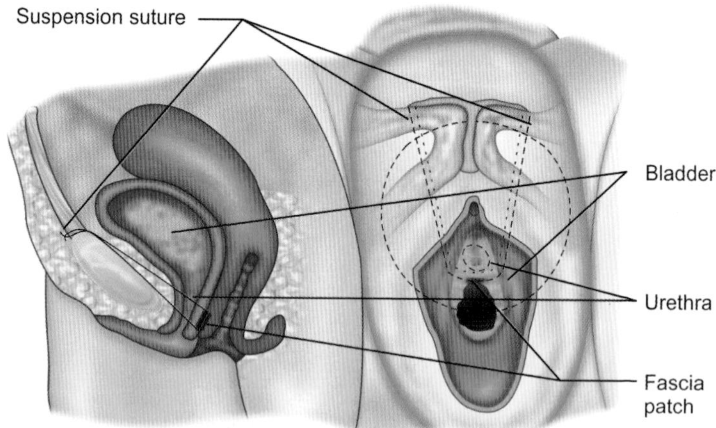

Figure 8.2: Rectus fascia or fascia lata suburethral (patch) sling. Prepare short strip of fascia from abdomen or from side of leg, place under bladder neck, and hang by suspension sutures tied over suprapubic area

incontinence after a synthetic sling or have had a complication after a synthetic sling such as vaginal erosion may be good candidates for a biologic sling.

Finally, we prefer to use a biologic sling in patients who have undergone radiation or who have had urethral injuries and patients who are undergoing either simultaneous or prior urethrovaginal fistula or diverticulum repair.

Sling Materials

Several different types of materials have been tried and investigated for use as a pubovaginal sling. The two most common autologous tissues are rectus abdominis fascia and fascia lata. Both have been extensively studied and have proven to be efficacious and reliable. Of the two, most surgeons prefer rectus abdominis fascia as an autologous material because it is easier and quicker to harvest.

Technique for Harvest of Rectus Fascia and Placement of Pubovaginal Sling

Technique

- *Regional anesthesia preferred*
- *Low lithotomy*
- *Pfannenstiel incision made, rectus fascia exposed*
- *8 × 2 cm fascial segment harvested*
- *Tension free suturing fascial defect*
- *Preparation of fascial sling*
- *Midline vertical incision at midurethral level*
- *Dessection laterally and anteriorly till endopelvic fascia*
- *Passage of retropubic needles with sling sutures*
- *Check cystoscopy*
- *Tension-free abdominal fixation to the rectus sheath*
- *Suturing of both the incisions*

- *Preoperative considerations:* Pubovaginal sling procedures are generally performed under general anesthesia, but spinal or epidural anesthesia is preferred. Perioperative antibiotics are usually administered with appropriate skin and vaginal floral coverage (e.g. a cephalosporin or fluoroquinolone). Antibiotic prophylaxis has now become a mandated quality of care measure in the United States.

- *Positioning:* The patient is placed in the low lithotomy position with legs in stirr-ups, and the abdomen and perineum are sterilely prepared and draped to provide access to the vagina and the lower abdomen. The bladder is drained with a Foley catheter. A weighted vaginal speculum is placed, and either lateral labial retraction sutures are placed or a self-retaining retractor system is employed to facilitate vaginal exposure.
- *Abdominal incision:* Transverse incision (**Figure 8.3**) is made 4 cm above pubic symphysis and the dissection is carried down to the level of the rectus fascia with a combination of electrocautery and blunt dissection, sweeping the fat and subcutaneous tissue clear of the rectus abdominus fascia.
- *Fascial harvest:* Harvest of the rectus abdominis fascia (**Figure 8.4**) can be carried out in a transverse or vertical orientation. Typically, a fascial segment measuring at least 8 cm in length and 1.5 to 2 cm in width is harvested. The fascial segment to be resected is delineated with a surgical marking pen or electrocautery and incised sharply with a scalpel, scissors, or electrocautery along the drawn lines **(Figure 8.5)**. Although virgin fascia is preferred, fibrotic rectus fascia can also be used. If resecting the fascia close and parallel to the symphysis pubis, it is advisable to leave at least 2 to 3 cm of fascia attached to the bone to facilitate closure and approximation to the superior fascial edge. Use of C-shaped retractor permits adequate retraction of skin edges, allowing access through a smaller skin incision.

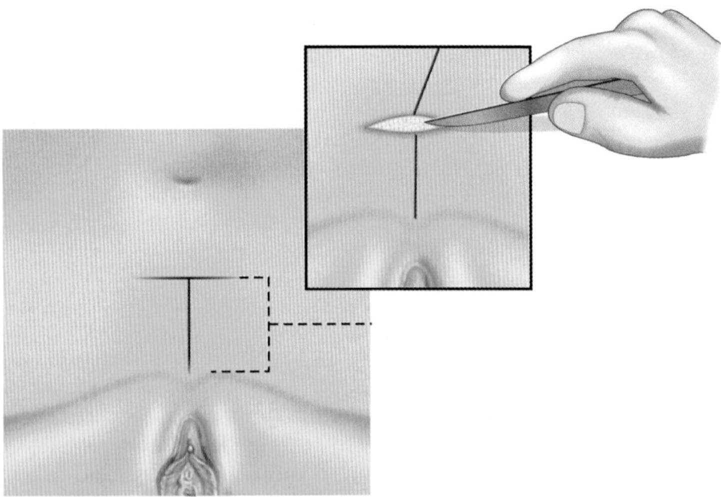

Figure 8.3: Transverse abdominal incision (4 cm above pubic symphysis)

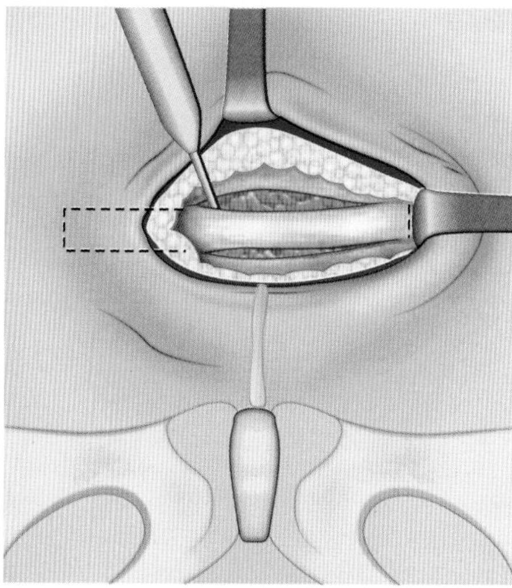

Figure 8.4: Strip of rectus fascia

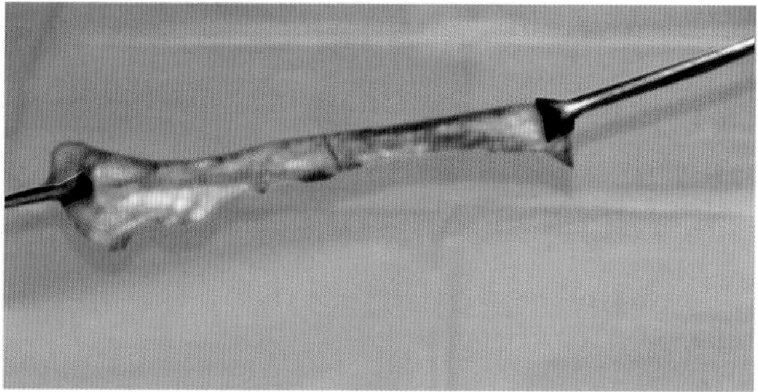

Figure 8.5: Pubovaginal sling of rectus fascia

- *Fascial defect closure:* The fascial defect is closed using a heavy gauge (No. 1), delayed absorbable suture in a running fashion. Mobilization of the rectus abdominis fascial edges may be required to ensure appropriate tension-free approximation. It is important to ensure adequate anesthesia with muscular relaxation or paralysis when the closure is being done.
- *Preparation of fascia:* To prepare the fascial sling for use, a No. 1 permanent (e.g. polypropylene) suture is affixed to each end using a figure-of-eight stitch to secure the suture to the sling. Defatting of the sling may be done if necessary **(Figures 8.6 and 8.7)**.

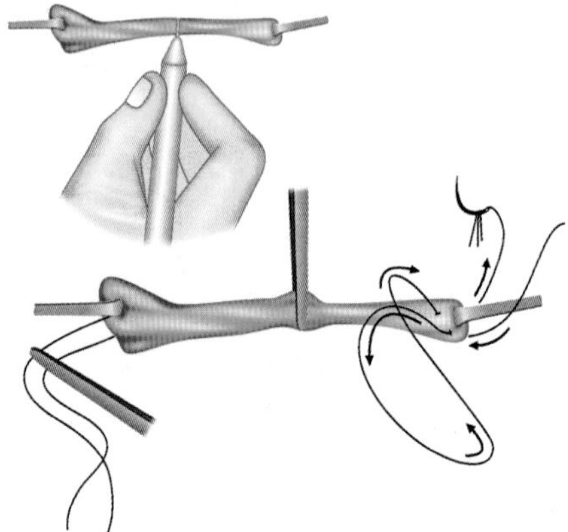

Figure 8.6: Preparation of fascia

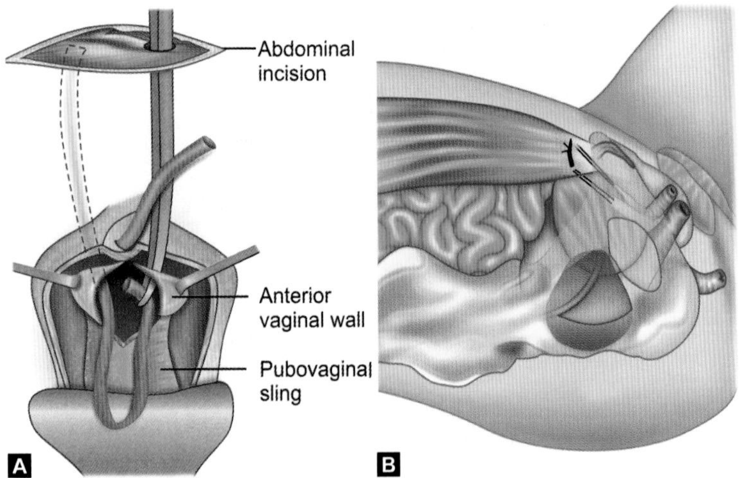

Figures 8.7A and B: Placement of pubovaginal sling

- *Vaginal dissection:* Vaginal dissection proceeds (**Figures 8.8A and B**) with a midline vertical incision. Saline or local analgesic, such as 1 percent lidocaine, may be used to hydrodissect the subepithelial tissues. Vaginal flaps are created with sufficient mobility to ensure tension-free closure over the sling. Dissection is carried laterally and anteriorly until the endopelvic fascia is encountered. The endopelvic fascia is incised and dissected from the posterior surface of the

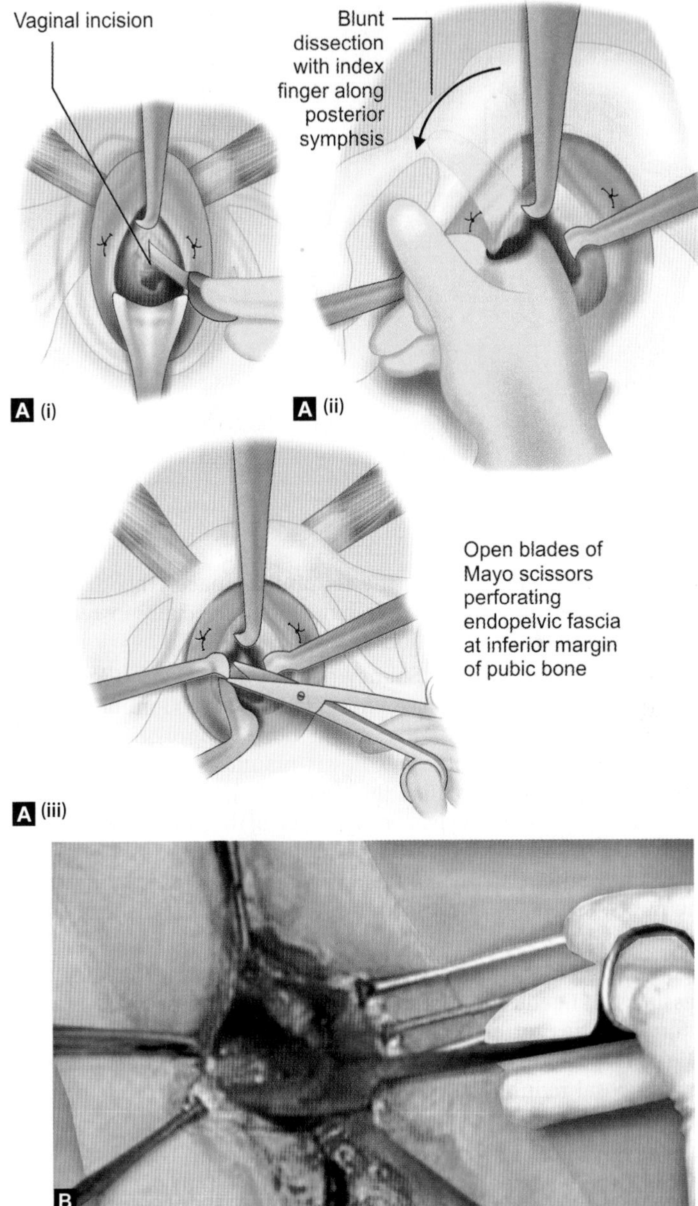

Figures 8.8A and B: Vaginal dissection

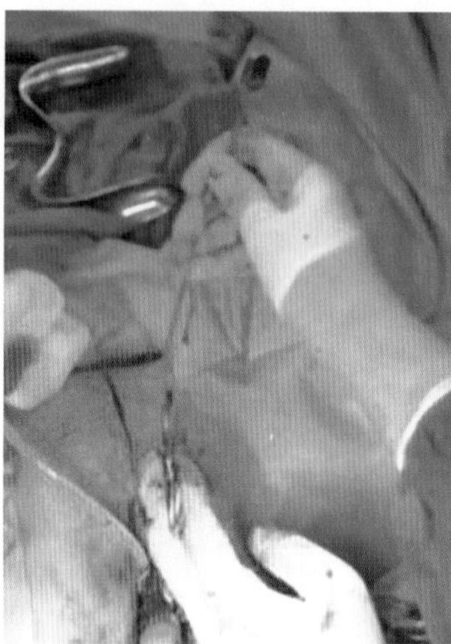

Figure 8.9: Passage of Stamey needle

pubis to allow entrance into the retropubic space. This dissection sometimes can be done bluntly but often, especially in recurrent cases, requires sharp dissection with Mayo scissors.

- *Passing retropubic needles:* Stamey needles are passed (**Figure 8.9**) through the retropubic space from the open abdominal wound immediately posterior to the pubic bone, approximately 4 cm apart. Distal control of the needles is maintained by direct finger guidance through the vaginal incision, and the tip of the needle is advanced adjacent to the posterior surface of the pubic bone to avoid inadvertent bladder injury. Proper bladder drainage must be ensured to minimize injury to the bladder, which may be closely adherent to the pubis, especially if a prior retropubic procedure, as in the case presented, has been performed.
- *Cystoscopy:* Careful cystoscopic examination of the bladder after passing the needles is mandatory to rule out inadvertent bladder injury. Injuries to the bladder typically occur at the 1 o'clock and 11 o'clock positions. The bladder must be completely filled to expand any mucosal redundancy. Movement of the needles or clamps can help to localize their position relative to the bladder wall.
- *Deploying:* To deploy the sling (**Figures 8.10A and B**), the free ends of the sutures affixed to the sling are threaded into the ends of the needles and each suture is pulled-up to the anterior abdominal wall through the retropubic space. Care is taken to maintain the

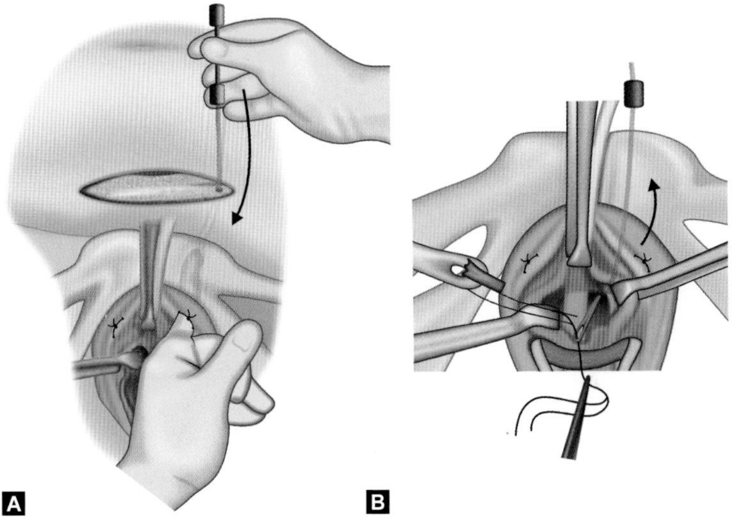

Figures 8.10A and B: Deploying of pubovaginal sling

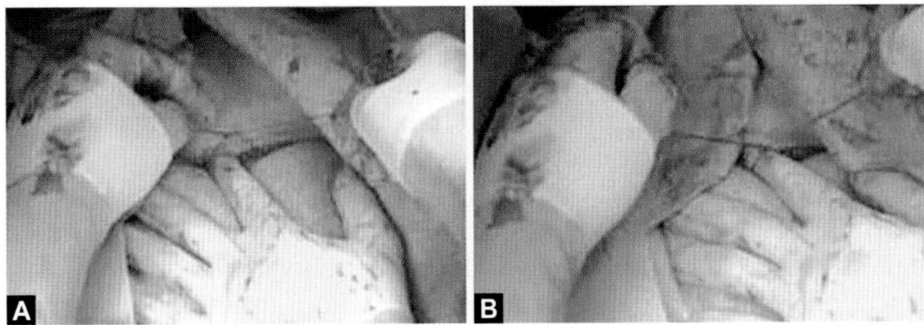

Figures 8.11A and B: Fixation of pubovaginal sling

orientation of the sling so that it is centered and flat at the bladder neck area. It is fixed to the rectus sheath.

- *Fixation:* Abdominal fixation (**Figures 8.11A and B**) is done by tying the two end threads together. Some surgeons prefer to fix the sling in the midline to the underlying periurethral tissue with numerous delayed absorbable sutures. However, we prefer to leave the sling unattached to the underlying urethra and bladder neck.
- *Tensioning of the sling:* Various techniques for tensioning of the sling are applicable. To ensure adequate "looseness," we prefer to tie the sutures across the midline while holding an artery forceps between the sling material and the posterior urethral surface (**Figures 8.12A and B**).

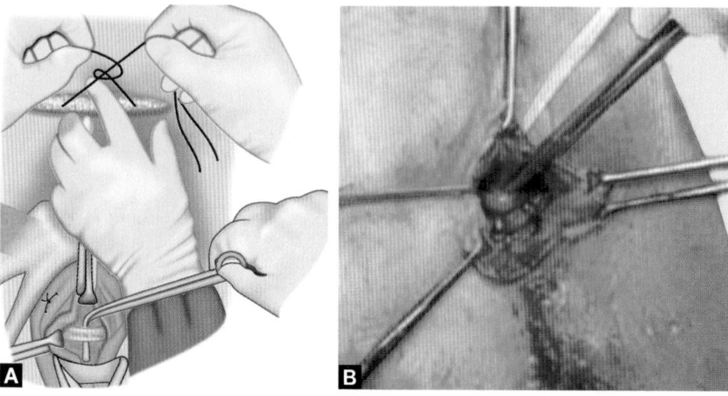

Figures 8.12A and B: Tensioning of pubovaginal sling

- *Suturing of both incisions:* The abdominal skin incision is sutured with 3-0 absorbable sutures. The vaginal mucosa is closed with 3-0 absorbable sutures.

A bladder catheter is left indwelling, and vaginal gauze packing is placed. The catheter and vaginal packing may be removed after 24 hours. If the patient is unable to void, she is taught intermittent self-catheterization or an indwelling Foley catheter is left in place for 1 week.

Autologous tissue from the iliotibial fascial band of the lateral thigh (fascia lata) has been used with great success as an alternative to abdominal rectus fascia for a pubovaginal sling. Although incurring morbidity of a secondary incision at a site remote from the abdomen, harvesting fascia lata may be suitable in patients in whom abdominal fascia may be of poor quality patients in whom extensive abdominal procedures have been previously performed, or patients with significant central obesity or a large pannus.

Harvest of fascia lata requires separate positioning, skin preparation, and sterile draping in addition to that for the vaginal procedure. To access the lateral aspect of the distal thigh, the leg is medially rotated and adducted. Two transverse incisions, approximately 5 to 6 cm in length, are made: a distal incision approximately 4 to 6 cm superior to the lateral femoral condyle and a proximal incision 8 cm cranially to the first. The incision is carried down through the fatty tissue to the level of the fascia, and the fascia is cleared either sharply or bluntly for an appropriate distance to attain a graft 8 cm × 2 cm in size. The fascial strip is harvested, using both incisions as needed for exposure. Once the graft is removed, the fascial defect is not repaired, and the subcutaneous tissue and skin are closed in multiple layers with absorbable suture. A drain can be secured in place through a separate stab incision and may be removed after 24 hours (**Figures 8.13 to 8.16**).

Outcomes

The literature shows that pubovaginal slings are highly effective with success rates of 50 to 75 percent when followed for 10 years (Norton and Brubaker 2006). In 2011, Blaivas and Chaikin reported 4-year follow-up with improvement or cure in 100 percent of patients with uncomplicated SUI and 93 percent in the more complicated cases. These authors reported that most failures were due to urge incontinence

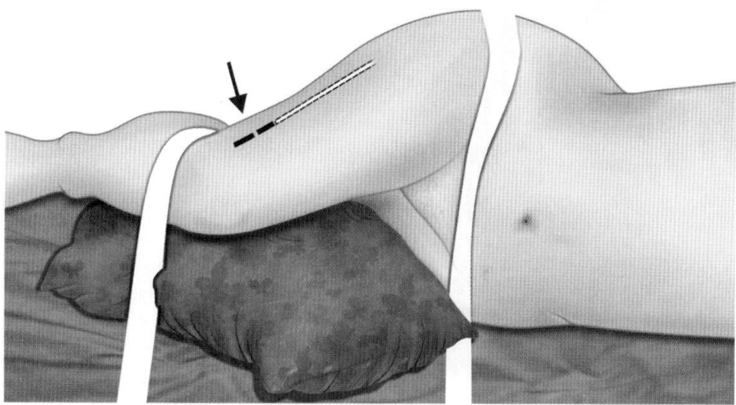

Figure 8.13: Positioning for excision of fascia lata strip

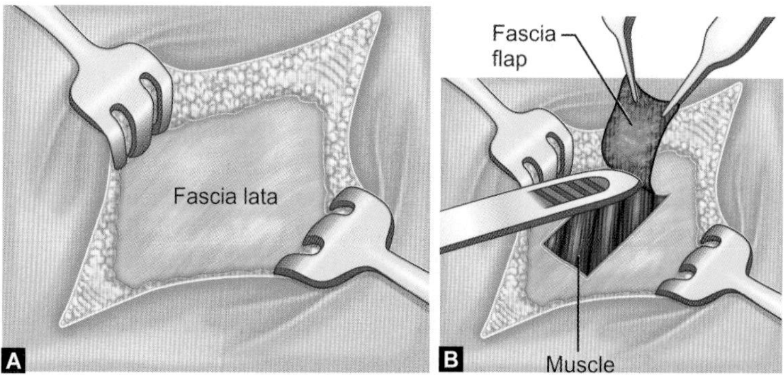

Figures 8.14A and B: Procedure for excision of fascia lata strip

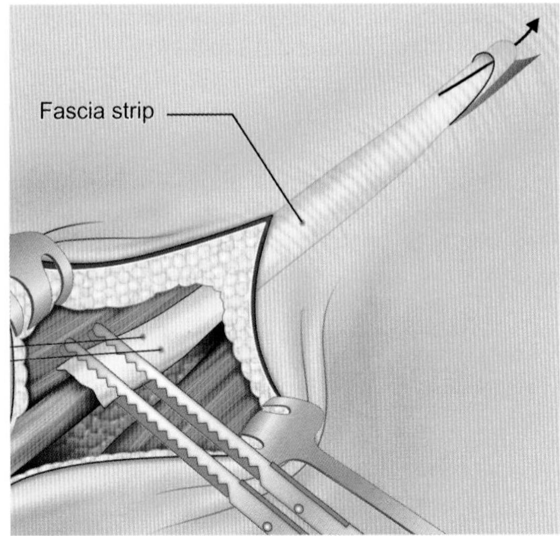

Figure 8.15: Use of fascial stripper

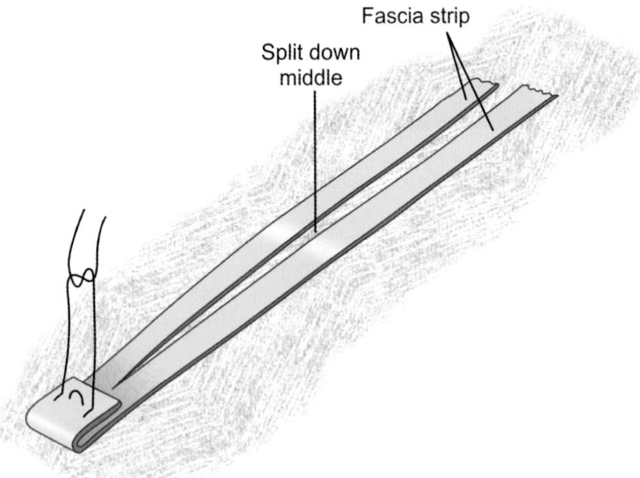

Figure 8.16: Fascia lata strip after excision

and occurred within the first 6 months postoperatively; 3 percent of patients with urge incontinence were believed to have developed *de novo* urge incontinence. Other studies reported development of *de novo* urgency and storage symptoms in 23 percent of patients with 11 percent of patients reporting voiding dysfunction and 7.8 percent requiring long-term self-catheterization (Norton and Brubaker 2006). The few randomized controlled trials comparing pubovaginal slings with TVT have had flawed methodology, and their outcomes are questionable (Novara et al. 2010). Basok et al. (2008) showed an increased rate of *de novo* urgency in the pubovaginal sling group compared with intravaginal slingplasty, whereas Sharifiaghdas and Mortazavi (2008) noted equal efficacy when they retrospectively compared an autologous pubovaginal sling to a retropubic synthetic midurethral sling. The most scientifically valid randomized controlled trial was by Arunkalaivanan in 2003, and it showed equal subjective cure rates and complication rates when a biologic pubovaginal sling was compared with TVT. In this study, the pubovaginal sling was of a porcine origin. When comparing autologous versus allograft slings, Flynn and Yap (2002) showed equal effectiveness in control of SUI over 2 years with reduced postoperative discomfort in the allograft group. Both groups had recurrent SUI develop in up to 10 percent of patients. Autologous pubovaginal slings were compared with Burch colposuspension in a multicenter randomized controlled trial (SISTEr Trial), noting superiority of fascial slings in controlling incontinence, despite an increased morbidity profile (Albo et al. 2007). In a meta-analysis in 2010, pubovaginal and midurethral synthetic slings were compared; equal subjective cure rates and equal overall effectiveness were reported (Novara et al. 2010).

Outcomes

- *Success rate 50–75% after 10 years follow-up*
- *Equal efficacy when compared autologous pubovaginal sling to a retropubic synthetic midurethral sling*
- *Pubovaginal slings compared with Burch colposuspension noted superiority of fascial slings in controlling incontinence, despite increased morbidity*

Complications

However, no surgery is without risk and the main potential complications are listed below:

- *Failure:* Most failures are due to urge in continence and occur within first 6 months postoperatively

- *Voiding dysfunction:* Transient urinary retention may occur in 20 percent of patients and requires intermittent self-catheterization until resolution (typically 2–4 weeks). Prolonged (persisting > 4 to 6 weeks) postoperative voiding dysfunction, including *de novo* urgency, urgency incontinence, or obstructive symptoms, may occur to some degree in 25 percent of patients. Less than 3 percent of women require subsequent urethrolysis for treatment of prolonged retention or obstructive voiding symptoms. We routinely teach patients intermittent self-catheterization in the preoperative period to facilitate its use, if necessary, postoperatively.

Complications

- *10–15% failure rate*
- *10–20% urinary retention*
- *10–25% bladder urgency and urge incontinence*
- *5% Wound/urinary tract infection*
- *<1% Bladder and urethral injuries*
- *<1% Pelvic visceral injury*

- *Needle bladder injuries:* If inadvertent bladder injury occurs (<1%), during retropubic passage of the needle and is recognized in a timely manner on cystoscopy, the needle can simply be withdrawn and passed again through the retropubic space, and the procedure can be continued as planned. An unrecognized bladder injury can result in serious complications related to foreign body reactions in the bladder, including suture and sling erosion into the bladder, stone formation, and voiding dysfunction.
- *Pelvic visceral injuries and blood loss:* Pelvic visceral injuries and pelvic hematomas are rare and can be avoided or minimized by adequate dissection of the endopelvic fascia and retropubic space and careful needle passage in close proximity to the posterior surface of the pubic bone with distal needle control with the surgeon's finger. If an inadvertent cystotomy or urethrotomy were to occur, the injury should be appropriately repaired. In contrast to synthetic sling placement, which would commonly require aborting the procedure, a biologic sling could still be placed after concurrent intraoperative repair of the injury.
- *Miscellaneous surgical complications:* Superficial wound infection, subcutaneous seromas and abdominal fascial hernias are uncommon. In obese patients, the use of a subcutaneous drain may be required to prevent fluid loculations.

- *Sling erosions:* Sling erosions with autologous tissue are exceedingly rare.

Key surgical points

- *Sling should be prepared before vaginal incision to avoid unnecessary bleeding*
- *In concurrent urethral reconstruction sling should be deployed and fixation is done after reconstruction*
- *Body side of the graft should be placed body side*
- *In multiple surgeries failure, sling tension should be significant*

Key Surgical Points

- Harvesting the autologous fascia and preparing the sling by affixing sutures should be performed first, before vaginal dissection, so that the sling may be inserted and deployed in a timely manner and blood loss can be minimized. Retropubic bleeding occurring during dissection almost always resolves with sling placement, and time should not be spent on prolonged attempts at hemostasis.
- When performing an autologous pubovaginal sling procedure in the setting of urethral reconstruction (e.g. urethrovaginal fistula or diverticulum resection) or as tissue interposition, harvesting fascia and preparing and deploying the sling with passage of the retropubic sutures, but not tensioning, should be performed before the delicate urethral reconstruction. When the reconstruction is finished, the sling can be affixed in the appropriate location and tensioned. Damage to the reconstruction can occur through traction or direct injury, if the sling is deployed after reconstruction.
- Surface orientation of the autologous sling material during placement of the graft does not matter; by convention, the body "side" or underside of the graft is placed on the body "side" of the patient.
- For most women, sling tensioning can be accomplished with the "two finger" distance over the fascia. However, in women who have had multiple procedures and have a nonmobile urethra, the sling tension should be more significant, using a one-fingerbreadth knot with concomitant cystoscopic evidence of an impression (lip or ledge) being created on the ventrum of the urethra.

As better insight into the relationship between the sling materials and the host response is elucidated, the success rates of sling surgery will continue to improve. At present, synthetic polypropylene mesh midurethral slings seem to have some of the best durability with the least problems; they will be hard to improve on in the future. Perhaps tissue engineering using autologous stem cells is the next step in the evolution of pubovaginal slings for definitive correction of female SUI.

Bibliography

1. Albo ME, Richer HE, Brubaker L, et al. Randomized trial of porcine dermal sling (Pelvicol implant) vs. tension-free vaginal tape (TVT) in the surgical treatment of stress urinary incontinence: a questionnaire based study. Int Urogynecol J Pelvic Floor Dysfunct. 2003;14:17-23.
2. Albo ME, Richter HE, Brubaker L, et al. Urinary Incontinence Treatment Network. Burch colposuspension versus fascial sling to reduce urinary stress incontinence. N Engl J Med. 2007;356(21):2143-55.
3. Arunkalaivanan AS, Barrington JW. Randomized trial of porcine dermal sling (Pelvicol implant) vs. tension-free vaginal tape (TVT) in the surgical treatment of stress incontinence: a questionnaire-based study. Int Urogynecol J Pelvic Floor Dysfunct. 2003;14(1):17-23.
4. Basok EK, Yildirim A, Atsu N, et al. Cadaveric fascia lata versus intravaginal slingplasty for the pubovaginal sling: surgical outcome, overall success and patient satisfaction rates. Urol Int. 2008;80:46-51.
5. Blaivas JG, Chaikin DC. Pubovaginal fascial sling for the treatment of all types of stress urinary incontinence: surgical technique and long-term outcome. Urol Clin North Am. 2011;38(1):7-15.
6. Blaivas JG, Olsson CS. Stress incontinence: classification and surgical approach. J Urol.1988;139:727-31.
7. Chaikin DC, Rosenthal J, Blaivas JG. Pubovaginal fascial sling for all types of stress urinary incontinence: long term analysis. J Urol. 1998; 160:1312-6.
8. Flynn BJ, Yap WT. Pubovaginal sling using allograft fascia lata versus autograft fascia for all types of stress urinary incontinence: 2-year minimum follow-up. J Urol. 2002;167(2 Pt 1):608-12.
9. Norton P, Brubaker L. Urinary incontinence in women. Lancet. 2006;367(9504):57-67.
10. Novara G, Artibani W, Barber MD, et al. Updated systematic review and meta-analysis of the comparative data on colposuspensions, pubovaginal slings, and midurethral tapes in the surgical treatment of female stress urinary incontinence. Eur Urol. 2010;58 (2):218-38.
11. Sharifiaghdas F, Mortazavi N. Tension-free vaginal tape and autologous rectus fascia pubovaginal sling for the treatment of urinary stress incontinence: a medium-term follow-up. Med Princ Pract. 2008;17(3):209-214.

CHAPTER

9

Laparoscopic Surgery for Urinary Incontinence

Prakash Trivedi, Animesh Gandhi, Sandeep Patil

A wide range of variety of surgeries is available for stress urinary incontinence (SUI), which always make a surgeon think about it. Better health care, longer life expectancy with emphasis on good quality of life has become important. Not just for the cosmetic benefits but other actual advantages, the last few decades has seen rapid progress and dissemination of advanced laparoscopic surgeries. Laparoscopy has not only touched every potential space like the space of Retzius, paravaginal, pararectal spaces, but have also identified significant defects or even potential defects which are now possible to be corrected by minimal access surgery surgeries.

This chapter aims at describing laparoscopic procedure for SUI and discusses our experience in these procedures over the years:

Laparoscopic Burch colposuspension (Laparoscopic Burch)	63
Only laparoscopic Burch colposuspension (Laparoscopic Burch)	43
Laparoscopic Burch with history of previous cesarean section	12
Laparoscopic Burch with laparoscopic hysterectomy	12
Laparoscopic Burch with vaginal hysterectomy	3
Posthysterectomy laparoscopic Burch	5
Laparoscopic Burch with enterocele repair	3
Laparoscopic Burch with previous attempts to correct SUI	8
Kelly's stitch	5
Needle suspension	2
MMK	1

Complications

Urinary bladder injury	1
Bleeding-significant (450 mL), with laparoscopic, hysterectomy	1
Conversion to laparotomy	0

Due to hemorrhage ____ 0
Due to bladder injury ____ 0
Due to inability to access ____ 0
Late/Delayed complication:
Hematoma/ Collection ____ 1
Retention of urine ____ Nil
Detrussor instability (DI) ____ 3
Increased frequency of urine ____ 1
Pain ____ 0
Tissue erosion ____ 0
Port site discharge for long duration ____ 1
(Laparoscopic supracervical hysterectomy with morcellation done from the same port, with laparoscopic Burch)

Failure

Immediate failure ____ 2
Delayed failure ____ 2

Details of surgery

Time required for the surgery ____ 65 minutes to 170 minutes (Average 90 minutes)
Suture material used ____ 95 percent cases Gore-Tex usually No 0 or No 2)
Four sutures ____ 12 percent
Two sutures ____ 88 percent (All are helical/double bite at paracolpos)

Discussion

Burch colposuspension is till date the most acceptable and very effective treatment modality for urethral hypermobility. It has to be confirmed that the patient is not suffering from detrussor instability and there is no element of ISD, because these factors certainly affect the results of the surgery.

Urodynamic study is mandatory before undertaking any operative measures.

Laparoscopic Burch colposuspension is the most ideal technique because it gives the same results as the open Burch colposuspension in expert's hands. The cure rate and the improvement are comparable with conventional Burch colposuspension **(Table 9.1)**. Though we admit that it is totally a skill dependent treatment modality and it takes a long-time to acquire the skill, we always feel that there is no shortcut to this procedure.

The long-term follow-up results of the surgery are more important. In our study we have 80 percent patients totally free from SUI till date. Ninety percent have occasional complaints of SUI but it is acceptable and they are happy with the results.

Burch colposuspension can treat SUI simultaneously with any other surgery for, e.g. laparoscopic hysterectomy, abdominal hysterectomy,

Table 9.1: Results—longest follow-up is of 6 years			
	1 year follow-up	*3 years follow-up*	*5 years follow-up*
Total improvement	86%	84%	80%
Improvement	7%	9%	9%
No cure or improvement	5%	3%	0%
SUI (Iatrogenic DI)	2%	2%	1%
Lost to follow-up	0%	2%	10%

and vaginal hysterectomy or of vault suspension surgery. We have performed laparoscopic Burch with laparoscopic hysterectomy in 12 patients and laparoscopic Burch with vaginal hysterectomy in 3 patients.

As the vaginal vault is pulled up and anteriorly and is hung from the Cooper's ligament, we always performed a proper McCall's culdoplasty before starting the Burch colposuspension to reduce iatrogenic posterior compartment defects which is 16 percent. We prefer to dissect the ureter properly along its pelvic course retroperitoneally. This minimizes the risk of ureters included in the suture or getting kinked resulting into ureteric obstruction, fistula formation and the other complications.

If there is no previous surgery along the bladder neck it is comfortable for a surgeon, but dissecting the urinary bladder in case of any previous SUI surgery or even any laparotomy involves a significant risk in itself. The adhesions formed because of previous surgery are totally unpredictable/erratic and at times can be significantly deep and thick. The blunt dissection of the bladder from the paracolpos may cause avulsion and significant thinning of the bladder wall with the risk of bladder perforation. We may have to shift to sharp dissection at some places.

As per our experience, the results of Tanagho's modification are significantly satisfactory.

Gore-Tex has proved itself as the ideal material for laparoscopic Burch suspension because of its unique quality of minimal memory and excellent sliding capacity.

In first 7 cases will used 4 sutures, 2 sutures on either side for colposuspension. But presently the same results are achieved with only 2 sutures, 1 on either side at the level of bladder neck but were helical or double bite at the paracolpos. At this juncture we want to emphasize that the results of colposuspension are totally skill dependent specially suturing.

Operative Steps (Figures 9.1 to 9.5)

In most of our cases we performed modified Burch's procedure. The procedure can be done by transperitoneal approach, which we do or can also be done with direct access to the retropubic space by an extraperitoneal approach. Transperitoneal approach allows simultaneous correction of enterocele and other incidental intraperitoneal pathology. In the transperitoneal approach we have the patient in modified lithotomy position under general anesthesia.

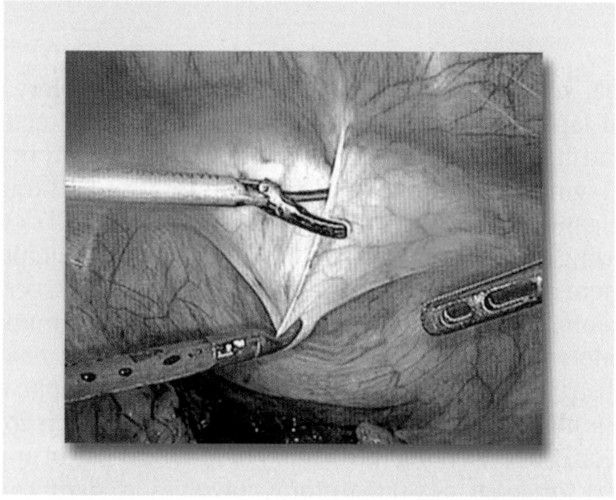

Figure 9.1: Median incision after filling bladder

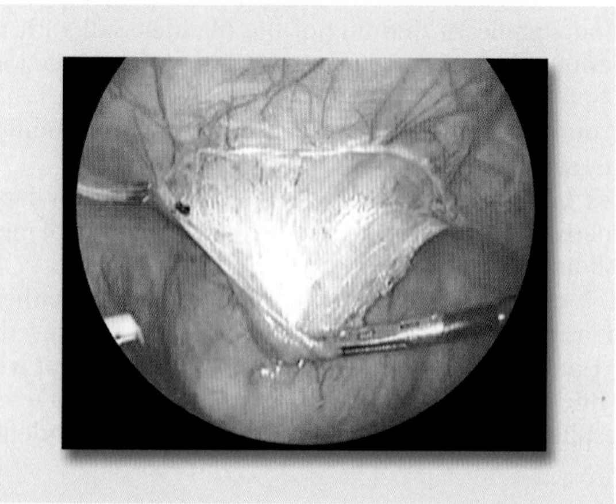

Figure 9.2: Horizontal incision between the two obliterated umbilical arteries

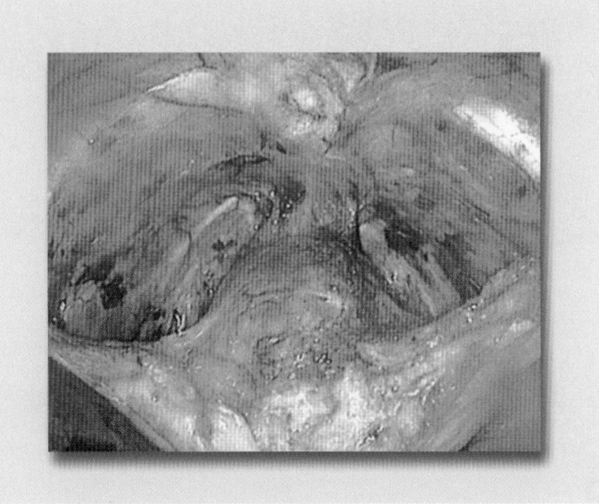

Figure 9.3: Space of Retzius dissected showing clearly the UV junction, left white line and the right shiny Cooper's ligament

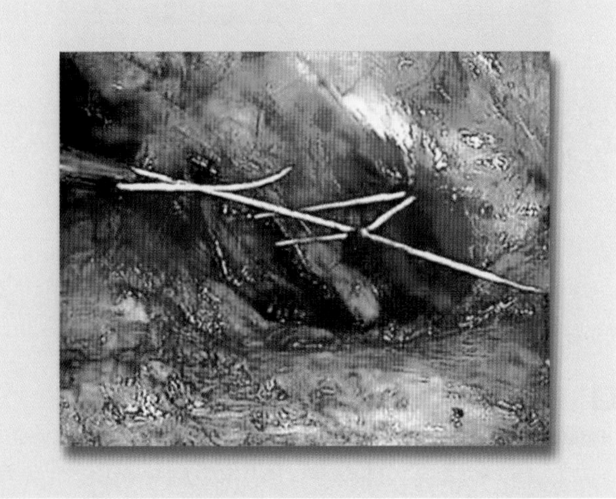

Figure 9.4: Helical suture being passed in right paracolpos and to right Cooper's ligament

The 10 mm zero degree laparoscope is introduced through the intraumbilical incision after CO_2 pneumoperitoneum created by the veress needle. Two ancillary ports are placed in the iliac fossa on either side lateral to the inferior epigastric vessels. Additional ports of 5 mm may be placed at higher level in the line with the umbilicus if necessary, more often on the left side lateral to epigastric vessels.

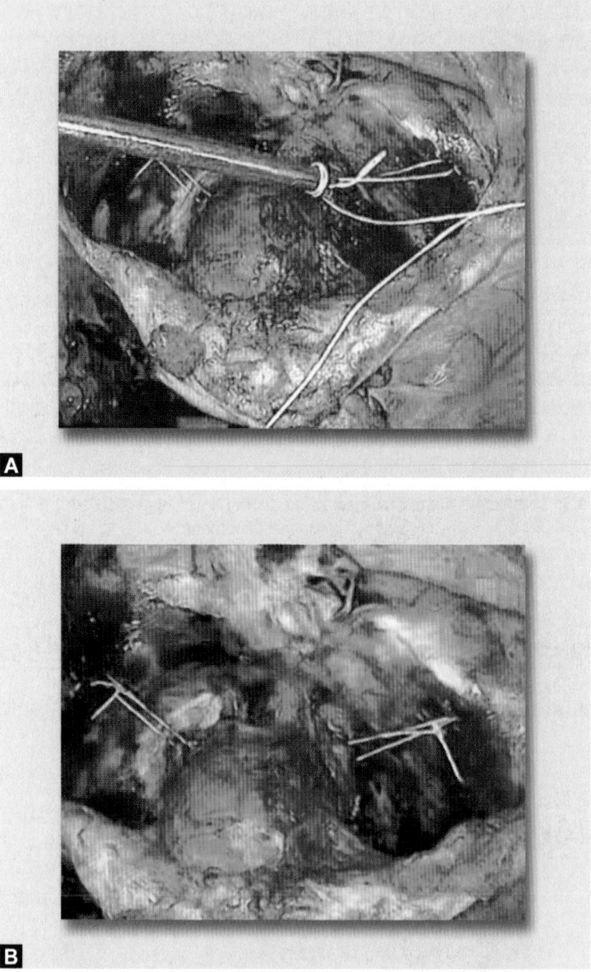

Figures 9.5A and B: Helical suturing being completed and space of Retzius: postcompletion of procedure

The urinary bladder is distended with 300 cc of normal saline or ringer lactate to identify limits of urinary bladder. The peritoneum anterior to bladder and 3 to 4 cm from the symphysis pubis is incised horizontally with monopolar current on a scissors extending laterally to easily identify the obturator neurovascular bundle on either side.

The loose areolar tissue and fats are dissected with gentle swipes with the back surface of scissors till the arcuate tendinous white line,

Cooper's ligament and paravaginal tissue is seen clearly. Bleeders are coagulated and one can identify the bladder with a distended Foley's catheter balloon at the bladder neck.

Once the space of Retzius is entered the bladder is emptied. Operator puts his finger in the vaginal fornix and pushes upwards the paravaginal tissue dissecting the bladder medially. Removal of fatty tissue in this area is very useful to have more fibrosis, which leads to better results in the procedure. Few operators do use a transvaginal illuminating device, which is not mandatory.

The first suture is taken 2 cm lateral to the midurethral segment taking the paravaginal tissue by a double bite and then passing through the Cooper's ligament. A number 2 Gore-Tex nonabsorbable suture with THX-26 needle is taken since it slides easily. The second suture is placed in similar fashion but at the UV angle, again 2 cm laterally and going through the Cooper's ligament but higher than the previous suture. Similar sutures are taken on both sides and extracorporeal suturing technique by our simplified knot and knot pusher is used to elevate the paravaginal tissue without much tension. Hence the suture remains like a hammock on either side. Paravaginal lateral defects are closed before Burch procedure, if present.

Cystoscopy in an occasional case is done to rule out inadvertent placement of sutures in the bladder and also confirming ureteral integrity with flow of Indigo carmine given intravenously along with furosimide.

Laparoscopic Repair of Enterocele

We always correct the enterocele before proceeding to Burch colposuspension. In most of the cases of laparoscopic hysterectomy we always perform McCall's culdoplasty, as many of the patients have enterocele or are prone to get the enterocele. The vaginal vault should be suspended with the uterosacral ligaments to prevent the vaginal vault prolapse in future. McCall's culdoplasty **(Figure 9.6)** or high McCall's culdoplasty is the preferable technique.

Ureteric dissection adds to the safety of the procedure and convenience to the suture placement. With the Gore-Tex CV2-THX suture material uterosacral ligament, the portion of vaginal wall, which is made prominent with CCL (Colpo Chirurgie Lausane) trocar in the posterior fornix vaginally, then the uterosacral ligament of the opposite side are included in the suture and extracorporeal knot is pushed with a knot pusher. Purse string suture including both the uterosacral ligament shortens the uterosacral ligaments as well as obliterates the Pouch of Douglas (POD). Care should be taken not to obliterate so much that sigmoid colon and rectum is obstructed.

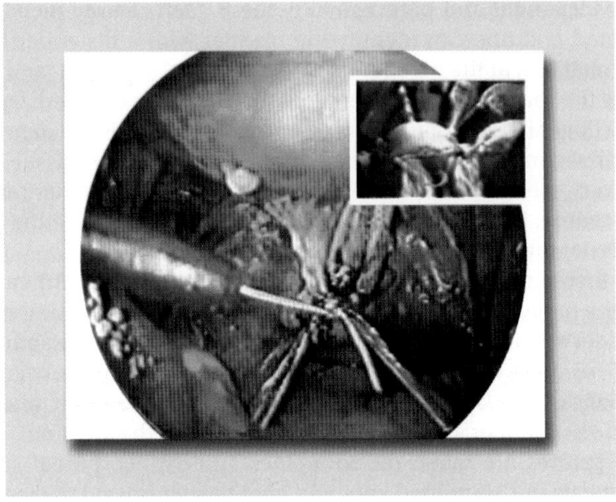

Figure 9.6: McCall's culdoplasty after Burch colposuspension

In our 63 cases of McCall's culdoplasty, we came to a conclusion that except the ureteric dissection the other steps in the surgery are easy to perform with good outcome.

Indwelling urethral catheter is passed. The ports are closed with 3-0 nonabsorbable sutures or skin glue.

The urethral catheter is removed in 36 to 48 hours and later voiding trials are performed within a week.

We do not put suprapubic catheter in any case of laparoscopic Burch colposuspension.

The procedure is not affected by history of previous cesarean section or even by presence or absence of uterus. However it is difficult if previous attempts have been made to correct SUI by conventional procedures particularly abdominal. We routinely take high McCall's culdoplasty stitch to prevent the future occurrence of posterior compartments defects.

Exposing 2 cm of paracolpos at the perfect site of suture placement, by pushing the urinary bladder from the vaginal wall demands great skill and good sense of laparoscopic surgery than dissecting and exposing the Cooper's ligament. Urinary bladder is filled with 250 mL of saline solution and the peritoneum incised 2 cm above the bladder margin. The cotton candy tissue in the retroperitoneum is dissected and Cooper's ligament is exposed at its thickest portion. With Cooper's ligament is located on the superomedial surface of the pubic ramus running from pubic tubercle laterally for 2 to 2½ inches. The exact placement of the suture is the key factor, which decides the result of the surgery. The dissection in the space of Retzius is limited to the aberrant obturator vessels. Variations in the Cooper's ligament should be noted. Sutures should pass through the paracolpos and then through the Cooper's ligament and should be suspending the paracolpos from the Cooper's ligament at least 1 cm distance to prevent the risk of postoperative urinary retention. The exact placement of the suture on the paracolpos is described classically as 1 cm laterally at the level of bladder neck. A Helical suture is placed on the paracolpos. It should be a deep suture reaching till the vaginal mucosal. Though ideally the suture should not pierce the vaginal wall through and through, it is not of much significance even if the suture is seen vaginally as it gets epithelialized. A deep bite through the thickest portion of the Cooper's ligament should be at least 2.5 to 3 cm from the midline. After putting the sutures on both the sides the hammock effect of the sutures is confirmed and extracorporeal knots are pushed followed by intracorporeal reinforcement.

The pneumoperitoneum exaggerates in the pelvic floor defects and similarly helps the dissection of "Space of Retzius".

Obviously there are the advantages of laparoscopy over the conventional open method as minimally invasive surgery, excellent magnification, tissue identification but still the comparable cure rates and quicker recovery. Better for concurrent posterior compartment defect correction or any other additional peritoneal disease of pathology.

More important in our scenario is that, the patient is not willing to reveal the problems due to SUI because of social reasons. It may be because it is linked to neurological incapability as in the infantile stage of life. Hence, the patients usually avoid a major surgery as open Burch colposuspension.

Complications associated with this surgery include urinary bladder injury as the most frequent complication. It is more common due to previous surgery and previous attempts of SUI correction. In our series we have come across 1-bladder injuries. At some moment we have felt the necessity of direct palpation of the tissue, which should have avoided the bladder injury.

With our overall experience and expertise of laparoscopic suturing we were able to complete the procedure laparoscopically by suturing the bladder. Laparotomy was not required in any case.

Occasionally we have come across the hemorrhage during the procedure but we have not faced the postoperative hematoma as yet. The intraoperative bleeding is because of the avulsion of the thin walled veins and it is important to know that use of bipolar or unipolar cautery is not many a times helpful, in fact it may worsen the situation. Pressure on the vessel can stop the bleeding even if it may stop on its own. Any collagen, e.g. surgical or any such hemostatic material may suffice at places. It is important for the surgeon to remember that getting panic at that moment may worsen the condition.

Essential 5 mm laparoscopic instruments for Burch or posterior compartment defect surgeries:

Long fenestrated grasper, Maryland dissector, disposable scissors, Robi bipolar (Storz), dedicated bipolar machine (Wolf), short flat forceps, short fenestrated grasper, specific set of needle holders Szabu Berci pair of parrot beak and Flamingo, long Scarfi's (Karl Storz) and long straight needle holder (Ethicon or creative surgicals).

Foley's Catheter Adaptor, Rectal Probe or CCL Trocar

Using current for dissecting the "cotton candy tissue" is useful as it prevents staining of the tissue and makes the tissue identification easier which is very important to prevent complications.

The dissection deeper is limited to the while line where we have to search for any breach in the white line, which is expressed as lateral cystocele during the clinical examination. This can be corrected at the same time by suturing the levator muscle to the white line. The bladder neck rests on the levator plate.

Though the detrusor instability is excluded before the surgery, it is not surprising to see the detrusor instability in postoperative period. This may be because DI is unmasked or exaggerated due to correction of urethral hypermobility or it may occur as an undesired hypersensitivity of the bladder to the procedure.

We have come across the postoperative urinary retention only in one patient. The hammock formed because of the suspending of the paracolpos to the Cooper's ligament is important and there is no role of direct compression of the bladder neck by the suture. The bladder is pushed down when the intra-abdominal pressure increases but the bladder neck and the uretherovesical junction is kept static due to colposuspension. The kinking of the urethra maintains the urinary continence.

Average duration for the surgery is 60 to 95 minutes in our hand (52 -170 minutes) during initial period or cases where previous surgical attempts were made particularly abdominal.

The laparoscopic surgeon should be well versed with different techniques of laparoscopic suturing, i.e. ipsilateral and contralateral, because the situation may at times demand for some on the spot modification in the technique.

After the surgery the patient is observed for 48 hours and the Foley's catheter is removed. On the next day the patient can be discharged after confirming the smooth recovery and normal bladder function.

CHAPTER

10

Synthetic Suburethral Slings

Prakash Trivedi, Animesh Gandhi, Sandeep Patil

Tension-free vaginal tape (TVT) is one of the minimally invasive devices invented, based on the suburethral sling theory. It is a logical extension of the ideology of supporting the vesicourethral junction at suburethral level in cases of stress urinary incontinence (SUI) due to both urethral hypermobility and intrinsic sphincter deficiency. Use of synthetic mesh instead of biologic material is used in the procedure.

Most important point about TVT is that, it is effective in both the types of SUI, i.e. urethral hypermobility and intrinsic sphincter deficiency.

Mechanism of action and indications are similar to suburethral biological slings and is explained in earlier in this book.

Procedure of Tension-free Vaginal Tape/ Trivedi's SUI Tape (TSUIT)

- *Preoperative considerations:* Pubovaginal sling procedures are generally performed under general anesthesia, but spinal or epidural anesthesia is preferred. Perioperative antibiotics are usually administered with appropriate skin and vaginal floral coverage (e.g. a cephalosporin or fluoroquinolone). Antibiotic prophylaxis has now become a mandated quality of care measure in the United States.
- *Positioning:* The patient is placed in the low lithotomy position with legs in stirrups, and the abdomen and perineum are sterilely prepared and draped to provide access to the vagina and the lower abdomen. The bladder is drained with a Foley catheter. A weighted vaginal speculum is placed, and either lateral labial retraction sutures are placed or a self-retaining retractor system, is employed to facilitate vaginal exposure.
- *Vaginal dissection:* Vaginal dissection proceeds with a midline vertical incision. Saline or local analgesic, such as 1 percent lidocaine,

may be used to hydrodissect the subepithelial tissues. Vaginal flaps are created with sufficient mobility to ensure tension-free closure over the sling. Dissection is carried laterally and anteriorly until the endopelvic fascia is encountered. The endopelvic fascia is incised and dissected from the posterior surface of the pubis to allow entrance into the retropubic space. This dissection sometimes can be done bluntly but often, especially in recurrent cases, requires sharp dissection with Mayo scissors.

- *Passing retropubic needles:* Use of a bladder manipulator passed via the Foley's catheter is used to deviate the bladder to the opposite side during passage of needles. Though the procedure is short, there is no place for haste during the procedure. The short distance that the needle has to cross should be actually felt by the surgeon keeping the attention at the tip of the trocar shaped needle. The tip should slide over the posterior surface of the pubic ramus and the needle should come out from the skin medial to the pubic tubercles about 3 cm lateral to the midline. This avoids injury to the lateral epigastric artery; obviously there will not be any risk of injury to obturator vessels. Raz/TSUIT needles can be used for the procedure. The major difference between the two needles is the thickness. While the TSUIT needle is 4 mm, the Raz needle is 10 mm. Obviously the track created by both needles is different and TSUIT needles offer a better grip within the tissues to the tape passed which is of 10 mm breadth.
- *Cystoscopy:* Careful cystoscopic examination of the bladder after passing the needles is mandatory to rule out inadvertent bladder injury. Injuries to the bladder typically occur at the 10 o'clock, 2 o'clock, 5 o'clock and 7 o'clock positions. The bladder must be completely filled to expand any mucosal redundancy. Movement of the needles or clamps can help to localize their position relative to the bladder wall.
- *Deploying:* To deploy the sling, the free ends of the sutures affixed to the sling are threaded into the ends of the needles and each suture is pulled up to the anterior abdominal wall through the retropubic space. Care is taken to maintain the orientation of the sling so that it is centered and flat at the bladder neck area.
- *Positioning:* The tightening of the TVT is not necessary. The artery forceps or any blunt instrument held between the TVT and the urethra in the midline at a slight inclination from vertical is sufficient and no more tightening is desired. As the procedure is done under local anesthesia, we can ask the patient to cough on the operation table and confirm the effectivity of the procedure. If the patient is sedated or under general anesthesia after filling the urinary bladder with saline solution, sudden suprapubic pressure is applied which acts as increased intra-abdominal pressure during sneezing or

coughing. One important test, which can predict the urinary retention in postoperative period, is to pass the lubricated Hegar's dilator in the urethra. Its easy passage through the urethra without any snap confirms the tension free position of the tape.

- *Closing the incision:* The vaginal mucosa is closed with 3-0 absorbable sutures. Abdominal skin incisions can be just covered with an adhesive sterile dressing or a simple suture can be taken in case of thicker needles.

Tension-free vaginal tape (TVT) however easy, it is a blind procedure. **Figures 10.1 to 10.6** can explain the insertion of the tension-free vaginal tape:

Advantages of TVT:
- It is easy
- Minimally invasive
- Effective for ISD as well as urethral hypermobility
- Less time consumption
- Minimal gadgets required
- Very short recovery period
- Can be done under local or regional anesthesia
- Very well accepted by the patient
- The effectivity can be demonstrated on the operation theater table during the procedure
- Suitable for the patients with any medical disorder or in cases where laparoscopy is contraindicated
- Anchoring of the TVT to the rectus sheath is not necessary

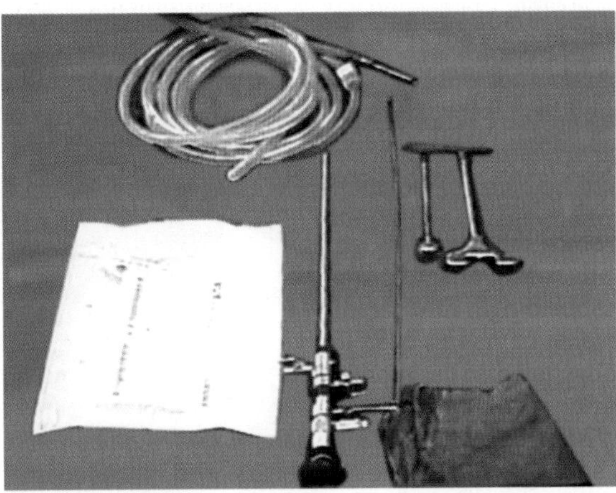

Figure 10.1: Tension-free vaginal tape—instruments

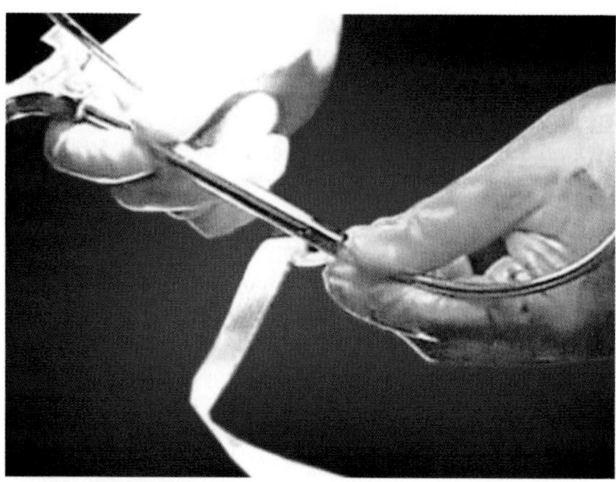

Figure 10.2: Tension-free vaginal tape—assembly

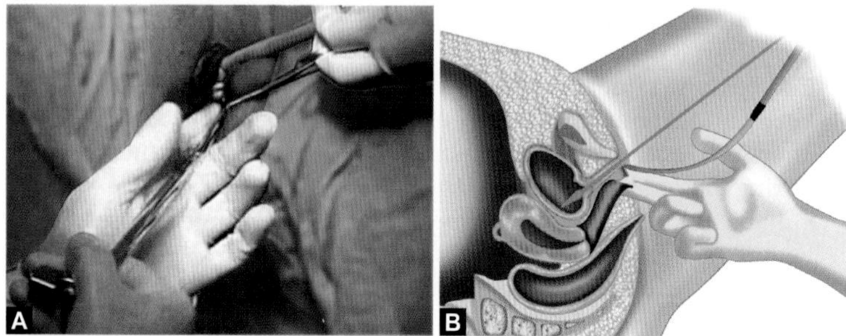

Figures 10.3A and B: (A) Insertion of the TVT on left side; (B) Insertion of the TVT on right side

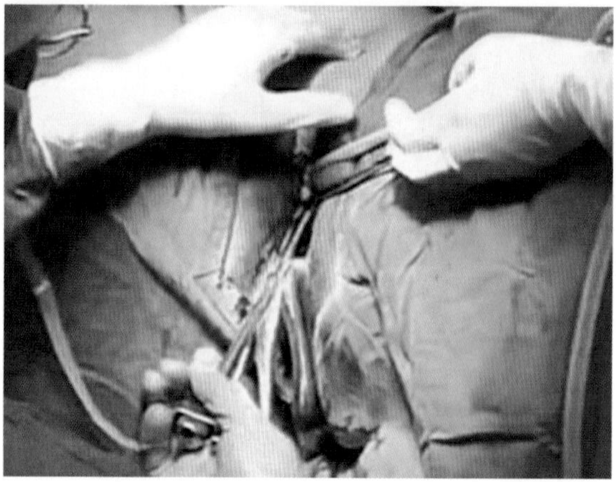

Figure 10.4: Insertion of the TVT on left side

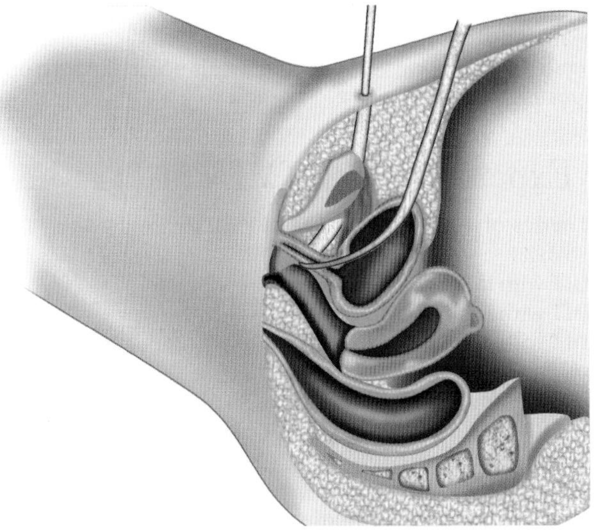

Figure 10.5: Confirming the tension-free application of the TVT

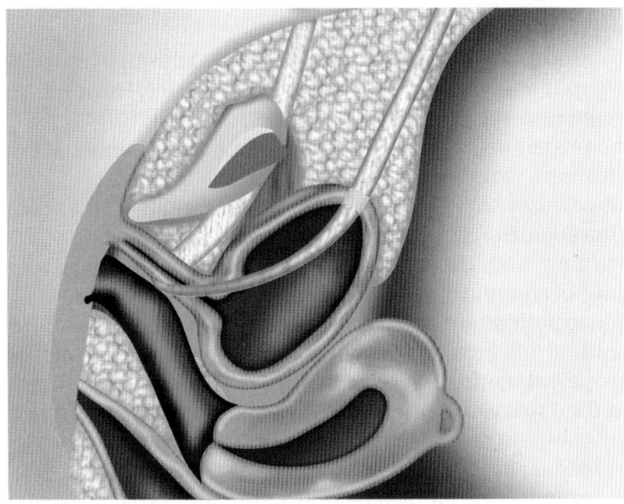

Figure 10.6: Midurethral application of tension-free tape

- Suitable for the patients with the history of previous laparotomy or any attempts of correction of SUI
- Overall learning curve is less difficult than laparoscopic Burch colposuspension.

Our Experience with TVT/TSUIT

In our series of 107 patients of TVT/TSUIT cases, 9 were TVT and 98 were TSUIT:

- TSUIT with laparoscopic hysterectomy 10
- TSUIT with vaginal hysterectomy 36
- TSUIT with previous failed transobturator tape (TOT) 5
- TSUIT only 43
- TVT with previous LSCS (Cesarean Section) 5
- TVT with previous attempts of SUI correction 4
  - Kelly's stitch 2
  - Burch colposuspension 0
  - Needle suspension techniques 2

96 patients are totally free from SUI. Maximum follow-up is less than 2 years.

We had to cut the tape due to retention or poor stream in 6 cases, out of which 5 cured and one has recurrence. Ten cases had perineal pain, which settled later on.

This procedure is apparently a real breakthrough especially for intrinsic sphincter deficiency or mixed incontinence. However, any tape is a foreign material.

The procedure is comfortable unless we come across the complications, which according to us are not infrequent.

Hysterectomy with TVT has less morbidity and less DI as compared to laparoscopic Burch.

According to our observation, patients, position also play a role in the incidence of complications of TVT, e.g. bladder perforation.

Bladder perforation is very common in TVT. In our series, we have apparently 6 bladder injuries. In 2 cases, the tape was not seen by cystoscope but there was a urine leakage from the skin incision and the paraurethral space. In 1 case there was a frank hematuria. In other cases, the tape was seen clearly passing through and through two walls of the urinary bladder at 10 o'clock position.

The common sites for bladder injury are 5 and 7 o'clock position and 10 and 2 o'clock position. Patients with previous surgery for SUI are more prone for bladder injury. A 70° cystoscope can easily detect the bladder injury. Otherwise, a cystoscopic skill is required to detect the bladder injury. According to the directions to use the TVT cystoscopy should be done every time after the needle peeps out from the skin. The needle should not be pulled out totally unless the safe passage both the needles is confirmed. Taking out the needle is too traumatic a procedure and can lacerate the urinary bladder.

In cases of injury, bladder catheterization was continued for 7 days and the patient's recovery was satisfactory.

The procedure can be repeated in the same sitting, but after second attempt we have to abandon the procedure.

Detrusor instability can be exaggerated after TVT, if close to the bladder wall. Though the bladder is not completely perforated, the TVT can include the bladder wall partially.

The bladder hypersensitivity is obvious with increased frequency of urine. It can cause an excruciating pain in the suprapubic region, even if she does not have urinary retention. All these conditions require medical therapy, which gives satisfactory relief but long-term results are still awaited.

There is a high-risk of erosion of vagina mucosal and exposure of the TVT tape to the external. The tape can cause erosion and visible inside the urethral canal. This risk of erosion is always associated with any foreign material grafts used during the surgery.

We have faced postoperative urinary retention in few cases and we have to cut the tape vaginally. In such cases, the tape should be cut on one side of the urethra. This relieves the urinary retention and still the urinary continence is maintained. The tape has specific structure that give the Velcro effect to the tape and the tape does not move or slip even after completely transected.

We have to modify the procedure in a patient when there was unavailability of the nondisposable components of the TVT.

The TVT can be used as procedure when TOT fails, or in cases of run-off incontinence wherein there is a leak of urine when patient suddenly stands from a sitting position.

The long-term results of the TVT are being published by many study groups and the results are satisfactory till now.

Average hospital stay after an uneventful TVT procedure is minimum 48 hours at our center, though shorter period of postoperative observation is sufficient.

This procedure seems very easy to perform but it should be taken up only after extensive training.

CHAPTER

11

Midurethral Transobturator Sling-Tape Techniques for Stress Urinary Incontinence Surgery

Prakash Trivedi, Animesh Gandhi, Yugali Warade

Introduction

Retropubic midurethral slings require blind passage of trocar through the retropubic space, inadvertent bladder injury occur in 3 to 5 percent of cases. Also, vascular and bowel injuries, though very rare, were reported that resulted in significant morbidity and mortality. In the hope of avoiding these complications, De Lorme designed the transobturator technique for midurethral sling placement in 2001.

Transobturator approach rather than a retropubic one, almost eliminates any potential for bowel or bladder and major vascular injury. Specially designed needles are passed either from the inner groin into the vaginal incision (outside-in technique) or from the vaginal incision into the inner groin (inside-out technique). When the procedure is performed in an appropriate fashion the needle and subsequently the slings pass through (from outside in) the subcutaneous fat, gracilis tendon, adductor brevis, obturator externus, obturator membrane and obturator internus. Transobturator tape (TOT) slings use the basic concept of midurethral support with the sling placed underneath the urethra; resistance against the urethra is generated when intra-abdominal pressure increases which increases outlet resistance and prevents stress urinary incontinence (SUI).

Transobturator tape slings are the most popular surgical treatment for SUI as it is a low risk procedure than comparable to most other surgical options in effectiveness.

Transobturator tape slings are associated with a lower risk of urethral obstruction, urinary retention and subsequent need for sling release compared with retropubic slings. For primary cases a TOT sling demonstrated similar rates of cure as compared to retropubic slings, with fewer bladder injuries or postoperative irritative voiding symptoms, major risk of bowel and major vessel injury are almost eliminated. The down side is that the patients experience more complications related to the groin, such as pain and leg weakness or numbness, with the TOT approach. Retropubic slings may be more effective for recurrent incontinence and in women with intrinsic sphincter deficiency (ISD), although the data supporting this statement are difficult to interpret owing to controversy regarding how best to define and diagnose ISD.

Numerous TOT slings are available at present time. Indications for TOT sling placement include patients with symptomatic SUI or missed incontinence in which the stress component is more severe than the urge component. TOT slings are also commonly placed in women undergoing repair of pelvic organ prolapse (POP). In the hope of preventing the *de novo* development of SUI (Occult SUI).

Primary Stress Urinary Incontinence

Surgical Technique

At the present time, the decision regarding which approach to use is based mostly on how a surgeon was initially trained to perform this procedures.

Inside-out Technique

The inside-out technique is of tension-free vaginal tape (TVT) Abbrevo (**Figure 11.1**). Transvaginal tension-free vaginal tape-obturator (TVT-O) is discontinued due to high incidence of the groin pain as the exit

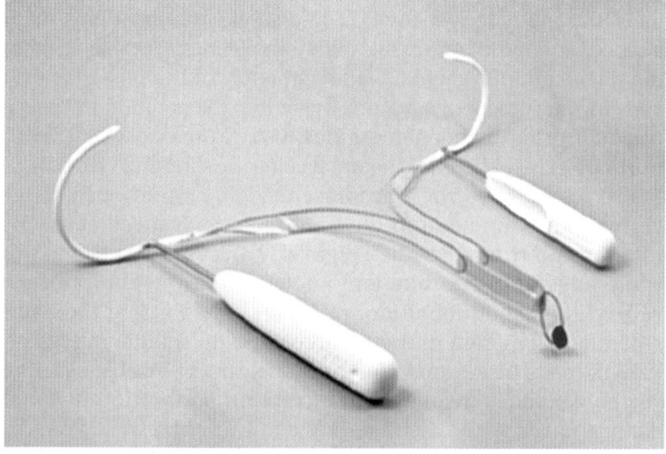

Figure 11.1: Tension-free vaginal tape (TVT) Abbrevo system

wound is close to pudendal nerve and tape being more porous attracts macrophages and inflammation.

Tension-free vaginal tape Abbrevo is designed like TVT-O but instead of tape there are removable threads at the exit wound. It also differs from earlier sling in that the sling is only 12 cm long (vs. traditional 20 cm long TOT sling). The shorter mesh traverses only the obturator internus, obturator membrane and obturator externus avoiding all the inner groin muscles.

- *Patient positioning and preparation*: The patient is positioned in dorsal lithotomy position with legs supported in Allen's or candy cane stirrups with all pressure points padded appropriately. The perineum and vagina are sterilely prepared and surgical draping is placed so as to allow access to vagina and inner groin.
- *Anesthesia*: Although the authors prefer to perform these procedures under low spinal or epidural anesthesia and local diluted saline adrenaline plus sensorcaine infiltration of vagina, which allows use of cough test to assist in appropriate tightening of the sling placement, can be also done under general anesthesia.
- The exit site of needle is marked. It should be 2 cm above the level of the urethra and 2 cm lateral to the labial fold.
- Vaginal incision, anterior retraction of vaginal mucosa with an Allis clamp facilitates visualization. We prefer to hydrodissection the anterior vaginal wall with a combination of adrenaline, sensorcaine and injectable grade saline. A scalpel blade is used to make a distal anterior vaginal wall incision.
- *Vaginal dissection*: Sharp dissection is used to mobilize the anterior vaginal wall off the underlying urethra. The authors refer to make the incision slightly longer for TOT and single incision slings than the incision required for retropubic midurethral slings. We prefer to mobilize the distal anterior vaginal wall completely of the posterior urethra allowing placement of surgeons finger into the paraurethral space for palpation of the inferior pubic ramus. Also we prefer to hydrodissect the trocar trajectory bilaterally before placing the sling and its trocar.
- *Trocar passage*: The trocar tip is inserted into the previously dissected vaginal incision lateral to the urethra and advanced gently while rotating the trocar handle (**Figure 11.2**). This insertion is done while hugging the pubic rami knowing that the obturator canal, which houses both obturator nerve and vessels, is at the opposite anterolateral margin of the foramen. The tip should emerge at the level of the exit site generated previously at the level of clitoris. The vaginal sulcus is inspected to ensure no perforation or mucosal damage has occurred. Certain sling kits (TVT Abbrevo) have a winged guide introducer that helps facilitate appropriate passage of the needle through the obturator membrane easily guiding the trocar into

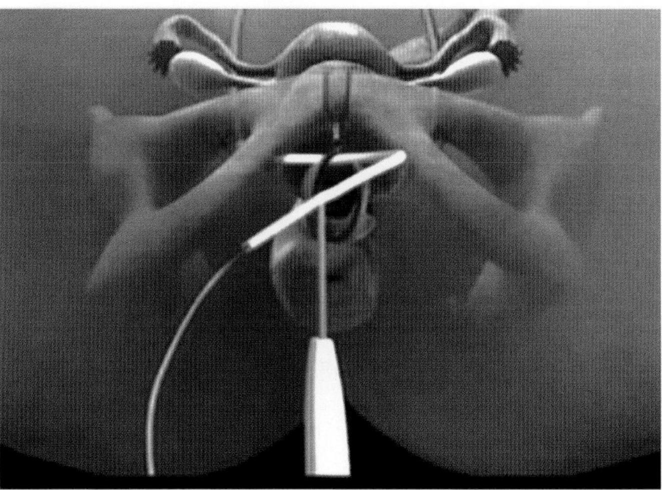

Figure 11.2: Right needle in vaginal incision

position (**Figures 11.3A and B**). Some surgeons prefer perforating the membrane with Metzenbaum scissors before passing the trocar. Once the membrane is penetrated with the tips of trocar, the surgeons hand is lowered or dropped toward the patient to allow the helical trocar to rotate around the ischial pubic ramus and exit in the inner thigh (**Figures 11.4A and B**).

- *Cystourethroscopy*: We do not do this in all cases except suspected or high risk for bladder injury. Careful cystoscopy of urethra and bladder should be performed to rule out bladder perforation. If the trocar were to perforate the bladder it would generally be visualized in the anterolateral aspect of the bladder (usually the area between 3 and 5° clock on the left side and 7 to 9° clock on the right side). If the trocar is seen in the bladder it should be withdrawn and reinserted. Occurrence of the bladder or urethral perforation or injury is extremely rare during TOT placement.
- *Sling tightness*: The sling should lay flat against the urethra easily allowing the passage of the right angle clamp between the sling and posterior urethra. We prefer to tension the TOT slings slightly tighter than retropubic midurethral slings (**Figure 11.5**).
- The vaginal wound is copiously irrigated and closed with a running no. 3-0 polyglycolic acid suture. The groin stab wound are closed with absorbable suture or covered with liquid tissue adhesive, this is not needed in our and few other techniques were the needles are only of 4 mm. If desired, a vaginal packing may be inserted temporarily at

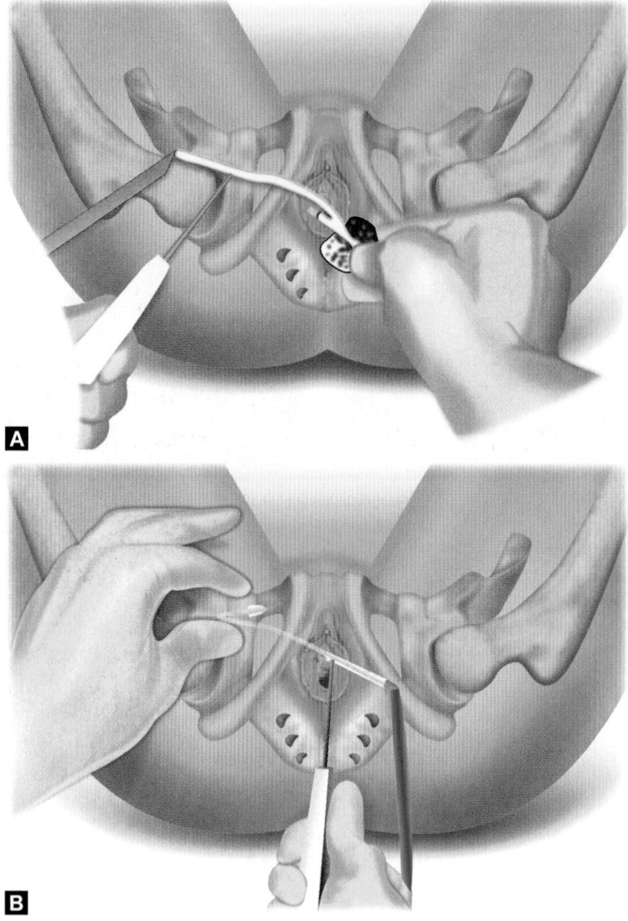

Figures 11.3A and B: Use of a winged guide

completion of the case (if patient is bleeding or concurrent prolapsed procedure is being performed).

10. The catheter is not compulsory, but if introduced may be removed (along with the vaginal packing, if present) in the recovery room, and the patient is discharged after documenting voiding efficiency. If unable to void, we do immediate postoperative loosening of the sling by urethral dilatation till 10 mm and also angulating the tip as it crosses urethra putting pressure on the sling which loosens, rarely the patient is taught intermittent self catheterization or an indwelling Foley's catheter is placed.

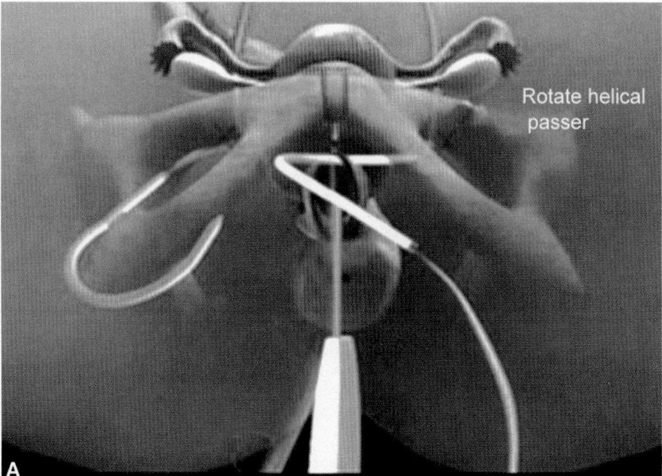

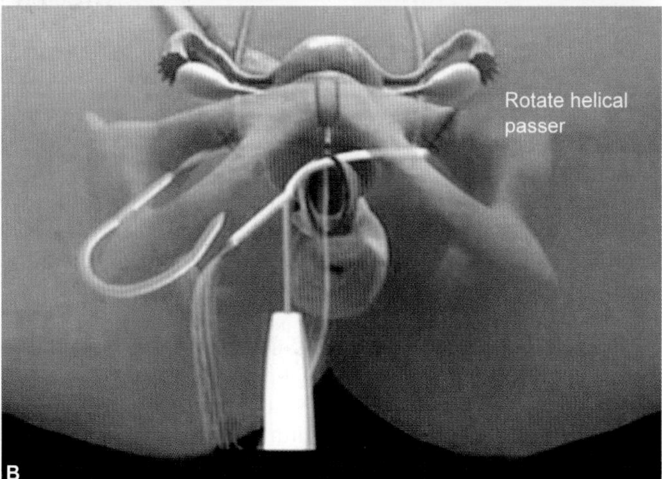

Figures 11.4A and B: Right tape passed, left being passed in helical direction

In TVT Abbrevo nonabsorbable polypropylene (Prolene) sutures are attached to the lateral edge of the mesh to allow for adjustment in mesh tensioning. Also, a midline prolene loop serves as a visual aid to help center the mesh. Both the loop and lateral sutures are removed after the sling is tensioned to the surgeon's satisfaction.

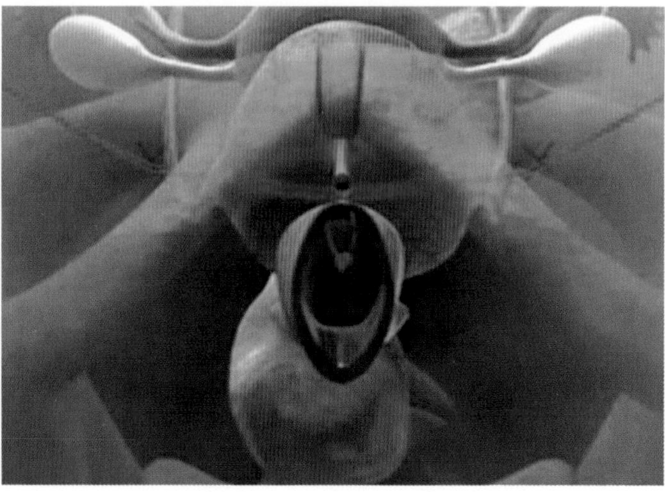

Figure 11.5: TVT Abbrevo in position

Outside-in Technique

- Preoperative considerations, patient positioning, and anesthesia are similar to inside-out technique.
- The penetration site for the trocar is marked in the inner groin, which should be just below the adductor longus tendon, at the level of clitoris 2 cm above the external urethral meatus. Local infiltration with 0.25/0.5 Sensorcaine is done and 4 mm stab incision is made in the crease of the thigh.
- *Vaginal incision* (**Figures 11.6A and B**): The incision is similar to the inside-out technique.
- *Vaginal dissection:* The dissection is carried laterally on both sides of the urethra aiming towards the obturator membrane. The incision should allow for passage of index finger to the level of inferior pubic ramus.
- *Needle passage:* We prefer to use Dr Trivedi's SUI needles and tape (**Figures 11.7A to C**). With the needle being nearly horizontal or parallel to the floor, the obturator membrane is pierced by pressure with thumb in vertical direction and the needle handle is rotated with handle at 45 degree and advanced along the ischipubic ramus with the needle exiting into the vaginal space previously created with the help of index finger as the guide for needle tip (**Figures 11.8 to 11.10**). The initial rotation should be to drop the handle so that it becomes perpendicular to the floor. At the same time, the trocar handle is dropped from the initial near-horizontal starting position to near-

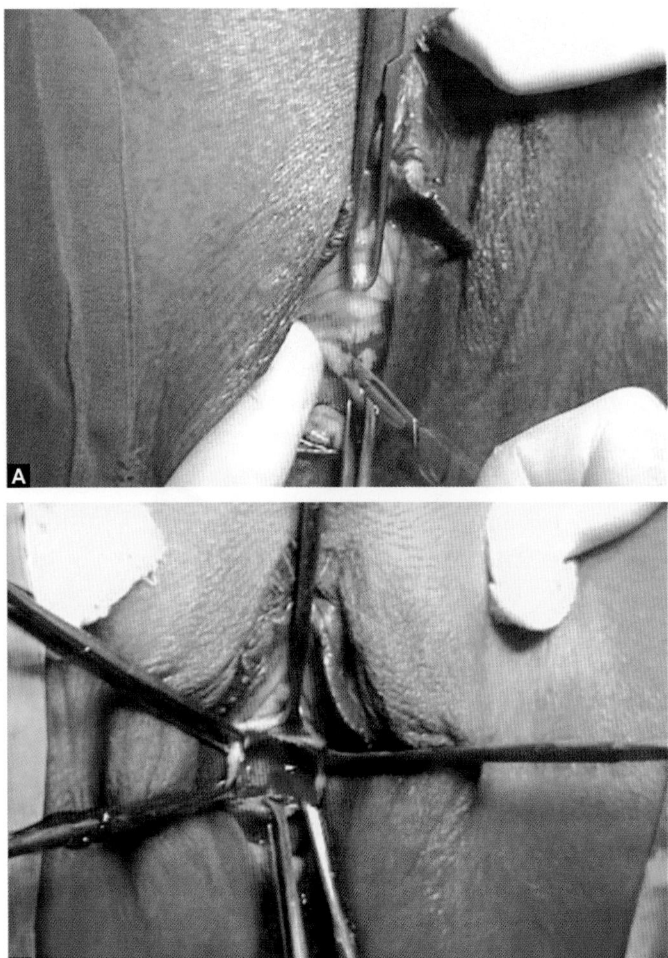

Figures 11.6A and B: Vertical vaginal incision

vertical position; careful angling and "walking-off" the bone allows for appropriate passage around the ischiopubic ramus.

- *Cystoscopy:* Rarely if needed cystourethroscopy is performed as previously described for inside-out technique.
- *Loading of the mesh:* The mesh is attached to the needle and the needles are withdrawn (**Figures 11.9A and B**), passing the sling under plastic sheath through the groin incision.

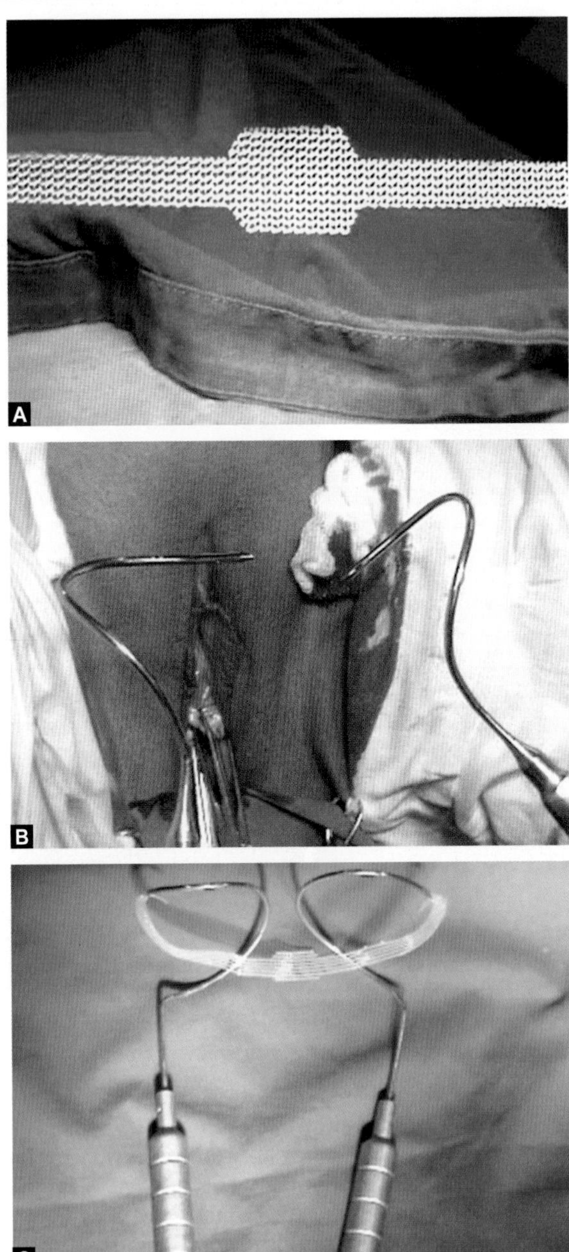

Figures 11.7A to C: Dr Trivedi's SUI tape and TOT needles

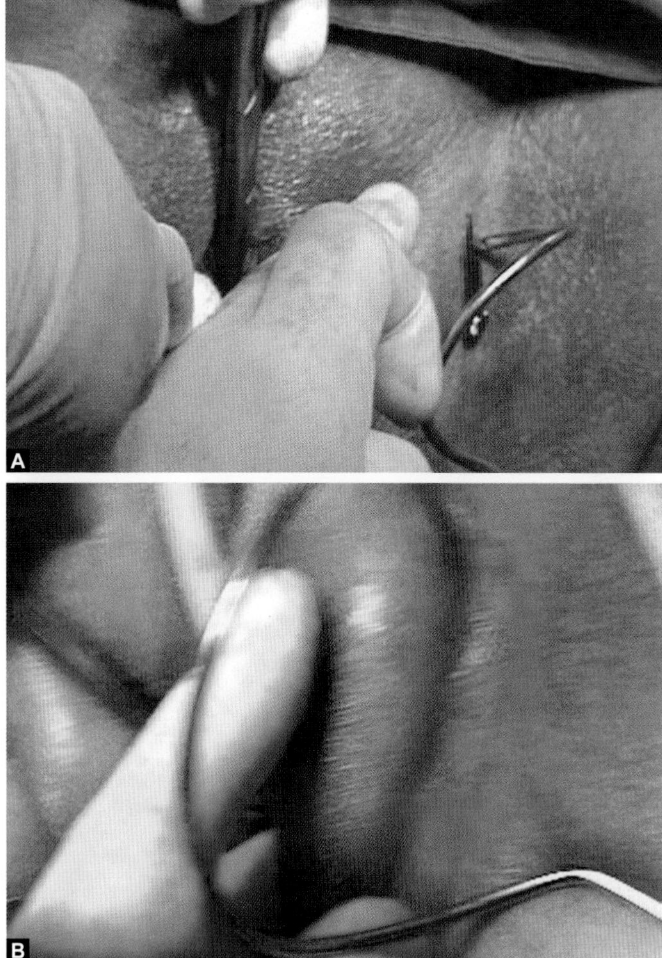

Figures 11.8A and B: Left needle passage in first vertical then at 45° angle

- *Tightening*: Tightening (**Figure 11.11**) is as described in inside-out section, using a long artery forceps.
- The wound is irrigated, and the mucosal edge is approximated using a running 3 to 0 polyglycolic suture. The groin stab wounds are not necessarily closed, if done with absorbable suture or liquid tissue adhesive.

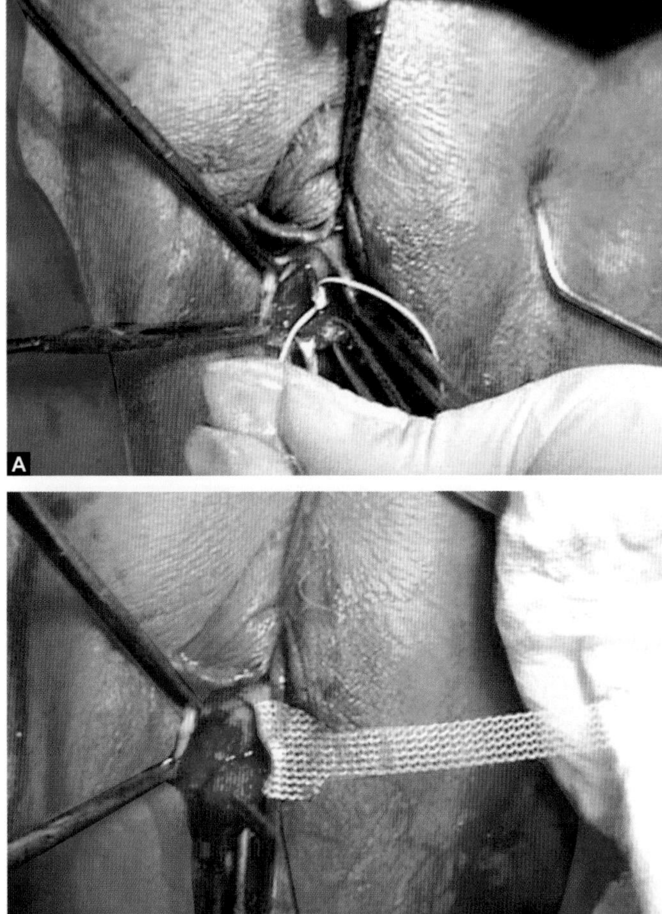

Figures 11.9A and B: Left part of tape being tied to needle tip and tape in place

- The catheter if passed may be removed in the recovery room and the patient is discharged after documenting voiding efficiency. If the patient is unable to void spontaneously, we do immediate post-operative loosening of the sling by urethral dilatation till 10 mm and also angulating the tip as it crosses urethra putting pressure on the sling which loosens, rarely intermittent self-catheterization is taught or the patient is discharged with the indwelling Foley's catheter.

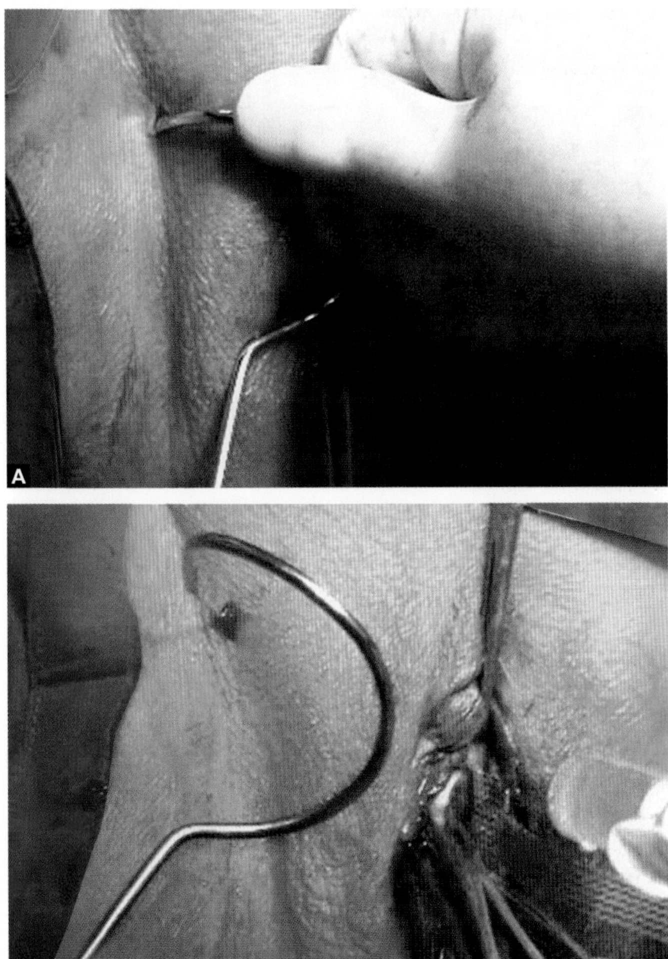

Figures 11.10A and B: Right needle passage: First vertical then at 45° angle

A specially designed Monarc/Dr Trivedi's needle is used for the outside-in technique of TOT. The Monarc needle is to be disposed but Trivedi's needle is reusable.

Many other methods are designed on a similar pattern. The new adjustable TOT (**Figure 11.12**) where a nonabsorbable threads are woven on the central part of the tape. Four threads go towards obturator foramen and four in the vagina. After the surgery till 72 to 96 hours if

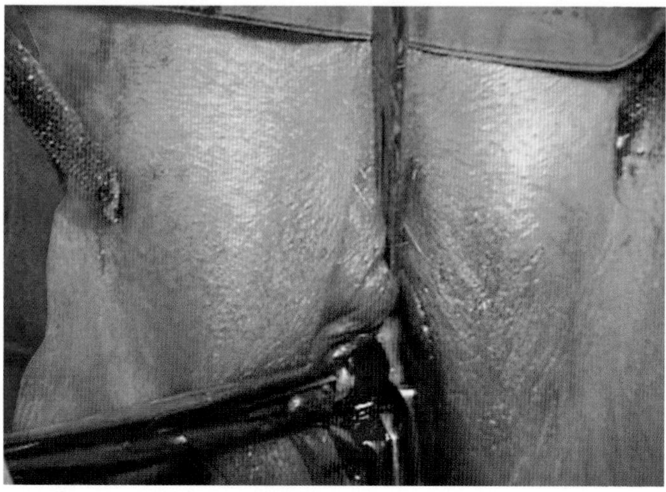

Figure 11.11: Final placement of both tape ends

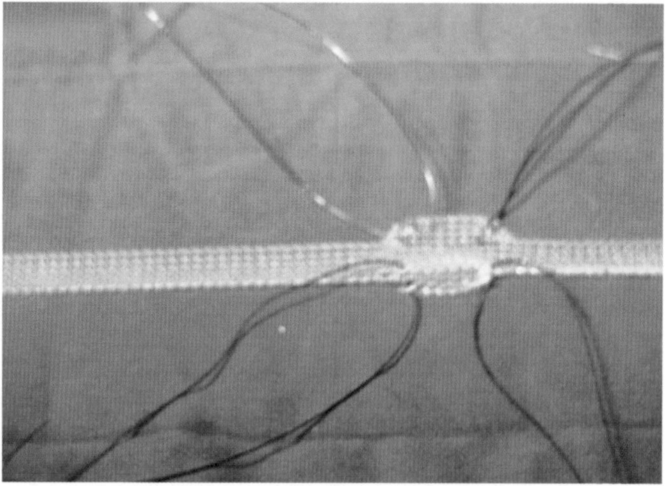

Figure 11.12: Dr Trivedi's adjustable SUI tape

there is poor result the threads in the obturator foramen can be pulled and if there is difficulty in passing urine pull lower vaginal threads; after which they can be easily removed by just by pulling one end of the thread.

Outcomes

A meta-analysis evaluating a phase 2 randomized control trial comparing retropubic and transobturator midurethral slings showed similar effectiveness in overall subjective outcomes. A Cochrane review concluded that there was no subjective difference in cure rate or improvement between the two routes. This conclusion was based on 10 trials involving 1281 patients. The same review reported a bladder perforation rate of 0.3 percent in TOT group vs 5.5 percent in retropubic group.

Outcomes of the two different placement techniques were evaluated in a meta analysis. No significant difference in subjective or objective SUI cure rates was observed. Also, there was no significant difference in the postoperative development of voiding difficulty or *de novo* urgency when the two techniques were compared. Outside-in technique was associated with higher vaginal angle mucosal tears during placement.

Intrinsic sphincter deficiency was shown to be an independent risk factor unsuccessful outcomes with TOT slings with an odds ratio of 1.9 favoring retropubic slings. Postoperative voiding dysfunction occurred less frequently in TOT group (4% vs 7% with relative risk 0.63).

Despite differences in technique and brand of mesh used, treatment success rates for uncomplicated primary SUI seem to be similar for retropubic and TOT tension-free slings. The percentage of patients treated successfully ranges from 60 to 96 percent (depending on how "cure" is defined). When the definition of success is restricted to SUI symptoms, especially over a short time, the reported effectiveness is high. In contrast, when the definition of success includes incontinence of any type, the reported effectiveness is lower. Retropubic slings, especially TVT, may be more effective for ISD, although this conclusion must be tempered by the small no. of studies addressing the issue and differences in diagnosis of ISD. Some studies have reported good success in treating mixed UI with the retropubic and TOT slings, although other studies have reported that the initial benefit for urgency or UI is not sustained over time, compared with benefit for SUI. It is important to counsel patients before surgery that improvement in SUI symptoms and general satisfaction is highly likely but perfect bladder is not.

Complications

Voiding Dysfunction

Of women undergoing TOT slings procedure, 4 to 8 percent develop some form of voiding dysfunction. Initial postoperative management includes catheterization; however, if this persists, the option of lysis should be contemplated. Urethral dilatation is typically not recommended because of fear of predisposing the patient to erosion of the sling material into the urethra, if done immediate postoperative period gently. *De novo* development of urgency or urge incontinence occurs in approximately 6 percent of women undergoing TOT sling procedures.

Groin Pain

Groin pain is reported to occur in 16 percent of patients after TOT procedures. The inside-out technique seems to be associated with more pain compared to outside-in technique. When postoperative groin pain occurs it usually is deep within the tissues and manifests when the patient abducts or adducts her legs. This pain is reported to be less common in patients who are overweight (BMI > 30). The motivation for development of the newer TVT Abbrevo sling was to prevent post-operative groin pain by not having any sling material present in inner groin muscles. In almost all cases the pain is self limited. In situation in which it is more sever or persistent, local injections of a long acting anesthetic in combination with a steroid may be attempted.The outside in techniques with 4 mm next and mesh which is less porous has least groin pain in obturator approach.

Dyspareunia

Dyspareunia is reported in 9 percent of cases. Slings which are palpable lead to dyspareunia. They are also predisposed to erosions. Excision of the palpable portion of the sling is usually curative of the dyspareunia but may rarely predispose to a recurrence of SUI.

Vaginal Mesh Erosion

It is a known complication associated with all types of synthetic slings. It occurs in up to 7 percent of women who have undergone a TOT sling procedure. Based on symptomatology and size and location of the erosion, appropriate management steps should be taken. This could involve simple observation in asymptomatic patient vs local estrogen cream vs attempts at mobilization of healthy vaginal wall over eroded tape vs complete excision of eroded tape.

Conclusion

With appropriate patient selection and placement, TOT slings have been shown to be very successful procedures for correction of SUI.

CHAPTER

12

Newer Small Slings for Stress Urinary Incontinence

Sarika Dodwani, Madhuri Gandhi, Prakash Trivedi

Introduction

In 2006, the single incision synthetic midurethral sling was introduced as modification to traditional retropubic and transobturator midurethral slings (MUS). These slings were designed to require less dissection in the midurethral area without the need to make additional incisions suprapubically or in the groin. They are placed entirely through an incision in the vagina having no exit point. They were designed to minimize the risk of bladder perforation associated with traditional retropubic MUS and the risk of groin discomfort or other issues related to the inner thigh associated with passage of transobturator slings through the obturator membrane and adductor compartment. Single incision mini slings are anchored into the obturator internus muscle or connective tissue of the endopelvic fascia of the retropubic space behind the pubic bone, depending on the configuration of the sling chosen by the surgeon. The US-FDA has required the manufacturers of single incision slings (SIS) to pursue additional studies to document long- term efficacy and safety further. These studies will be ongoing over the next two years and will determine the future of these devices.

Indications and Patient Selection

They are similar to the indications for the more traditional MUS. Because they avoid the retropubic space, the mini sling may be considered specifically in patients who have undergone previous retropubic and abdominal procedures and may be at higher risk for significant pelvic adhesions. Because it does not involve complete passage of trocar to the skin level, it may be considered in patients with significant soft tissue mass or obesity in the areas of tradition MUS trocar site exit (i.e. truncal or global obesity) that may surpass the length of the trocar. Because single incision mini sling procedure can be done under local anesthesia, they can also be considered in patients with significant comorbidities in which general anesthesia is contraindicated. At the present time, it is rarely used in patients with primary SUI because long-term data show efficacy comparable to retropubic or transobturator MUS are lacking.

Description of Various Types of Single Incision Slings

Five types are commercially available at present time in USA: TVT-Secur, MiniArc single incision sling system, Solyx SIS system, AJUST (adjustable single incision sling) and mini-tape.

The TVT-Secur is a preassembled polypropylene woven mesh tape (8 cm × 1.1 cm) and metal inserter device. Sandwiching each end of the tape are polyglactin 910 (vicryl) and polydioxanone (PDS) woven fleece patches that are designed to allow connected tissue ingrowth while undergoing concurrent absorption (within 90 to 180 days) encouraging the permanent fixation of the mesh sling. The sling and the inserter device are inserted and the position of the sling is confirmed after which the inserter device is disengaged and removed, leaving the mesh behind.

The MiniArc single incision sling is polypropylene mesh (8.5 cm × 1.1 cm) with permanent self fixating tips that is deployed with a supplied metal 2.3 mm needle/trocar. The mesh is connected to the tip of needle before insertion; the mesh and needle are inserted and the needle is removed, leaving the mesh behind. Self fixating tips are constructed of polypropylene and have two anchoring barbs that help resist up to 5.5 lb of pull out force to remove the mesh. A redocking maneuver can be set-up before inserting to allow retrieval and reinsertion of the mesh if necessary.

The Solyx-SIS system includes a polypropylene mesh tape (9 cm in length) with permanent barbed self-fixating tips and a metal and plastic delivery device or trocar. These system is designed similarly to the MiniArc single incision sling system, in that each tip of the sling is sequentially attached to the end of the deliver device for mesh placement, which is removed after insertion. The edges of the center 4 cm of the mesh (advertised as the suburethral portion) are bonded together to potentially of mesh erosion or extrusion.

The AJUST adjustable single incision sling is a new adjustable mini sling that allows the surgeon to tighten or loosen the sling after it has been anchored into the obturator membrane.

Stress urinary incontinence in a patient with significant comorbidities—Severe obesity.

Surgical Techniques

TVT-Secur

1. *Preoperative considerations:* Insertion of a mini sling may be performed under many different types of anesthesia, including general, spinal or epidural, regional, and local. Preoperative antibiotics are generally administered before the incision.
2. *Patient positioning:* The patient is positioned in the dorsal lithotomy position with legs in stirrups. The perineum and vagina are sterilely prepared and draped so as to exclude the anus. Lateral labia majora retraction stitches may be placed or self-retaining may be used to improve vaginal exposure. A weighted vaginal speculum is placed, and bladder drainage is accomplished with a Foley's catheter.
3. *Vaginal incision:* A 1 to 1.5 cm midline incision is marked starting 1 cm below the urethral meatus, and the area is infiltrated with injectable grade saline with 0.5 percent sensorcaine with diluted adrenaline for hydrodissection of the periurethral tissues. An allis clamp may be placed distal to the incision, with care taken not to traumatize the urethral meatus, to facilitate visualization. An incision is made sharply with a scalpel (**Figure 12.1**).
4. *Vaginal flap dissection:* Dissection of lateral vaginal flaps proceeds in a standard fashion with attention to developing an appropriately robust and well-vascularized vaginal flap, while not jeopardizing

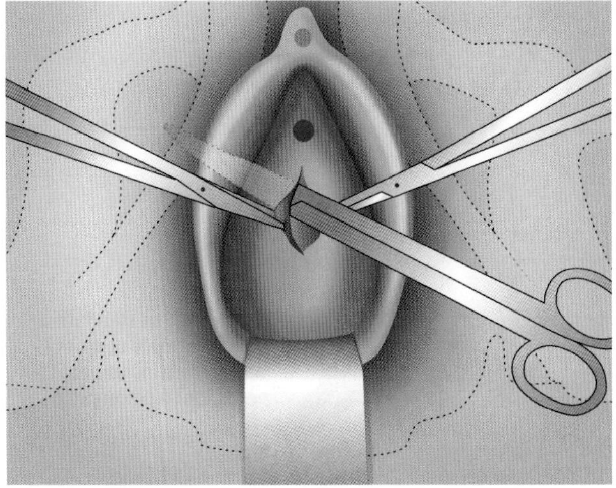

Figure 12.1: Incision and dissection of vaginal flaps

the thickness of the periurethral tissue. This flap is carried laterally and anteriorly, until the endopelvic fascia is encountered, but the retropubic space is not entered.

5. *Preparation of sling (TVT-Secur):* The sling is prepared by soaking in saline mixed with antibiotic. When ready to use a stout, medium length needle driver is attached to 1 of the metal arms of the device (**Figure 12.2**). This driver is used to assist in placement and to protect the disengagement pin.
6. *Configuration of sling placement:* The sling may be placed in either of the two angle configurations that mimic the angles of support achieved by either a transobturator or retropubic MUS. Inserting a device at a 90 degree angle to the sagittal midline achieves the angle of support similar to a transobturator sling, or what has been termed the "hammock" configuration. Angling at 45 degrees from the sagittal midline achieves the angle of support similar to the retropubic sling, or what has been termed the "U" configuration.
7. *Insertion of sling (**Figure 12.3**):* To place the TVT-Secur, the tip of the inserter (without the protective cap) is positioned in the previously dissected periurethral space, angling toward in the ipsilateral shoulder for the "U" configuration or toward the 9 o'clock or 3 o'clock position for the hammock configuration, and gently inserted until resistance from the pubic bone is met (no more than 3 to 4 cm). The inserter is slightly withdrawn, angled more posteriorly, and reinserted to "walk-off" the pubic bone. When the posterior edge of the bone is

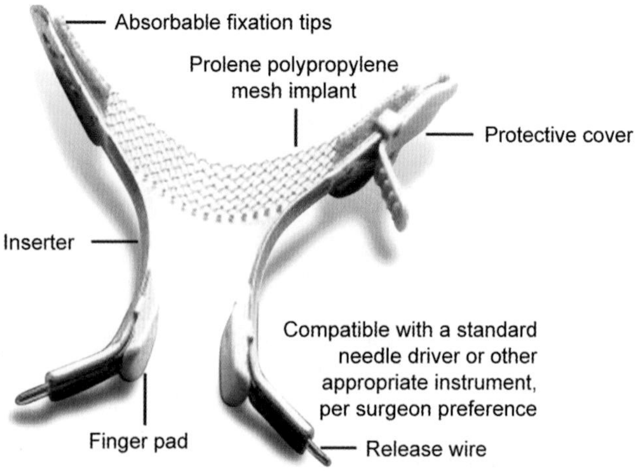

Figure 12.2: Tape with inserter

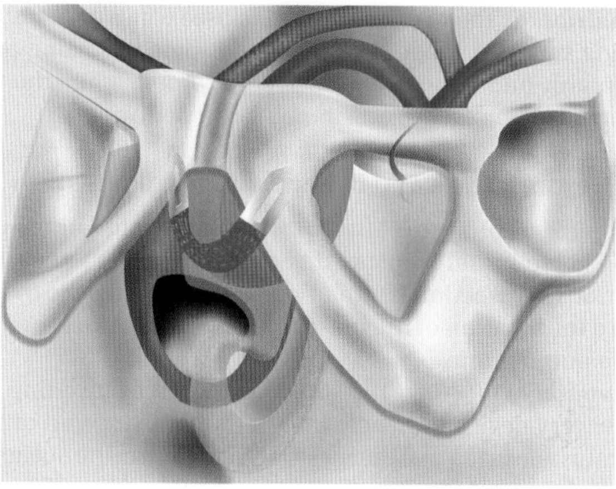

Figure 12.3: Placement of mesh

encountered (noted by a loss of resistance), the inserter is gently driven along the posterior surface of the bone into the connective tissue of the urogenital diaphragm. Maintaining close contact with the posterior surface of pubic bone minimizes chance of injury to pelvic structures; this is facilitated by rotating the device as it is advanced with the index finger applying pressure on the finger pad of inserter arm and lowering the needle driver towards the floor. When the inserter is firmly embedded in the connective tissue, insertion is stopped, the needle driver is removed and replaced to the contralateral inserter arm, and the maneuver is repeated on the other side.

8. *Cystoscopy:* Cystoscopy is performed to evaluate a bladder injury. The bladder must be completely filled and examined in its entirety with a 30 or 70 degree lens or both. If a trocar injury occurs, it is typically located at the posterior lateral aspect of the bladder base. Gently wiggling the inserter arms under cystoscopic guidance shows their location relative to the bladder mucosa.
9. *Tensioning:* The tension of the sling may be assessed by gently inserting an angled clamp between the mesh and the urethra. An appropriate amount of tension in the sling permits just the insertion of the tip of the clamp but not more. If the sling is deemed either too loose or too tight, it can either be inserted further or can be gently retracted, always moving the inserter arm and not the mesh directly.
10. *Deploying and disengaging blade:* To deploy the mesh sling and disengage the inserter arm, the release wire is pulled to the stop position while stabilizing the inserter; the inserter is withdrawn with a gentle twisting motion. This is repeated for the other side.

11. *Vaginal closure:* The vaginal incision is closed with a no. 2-0 absorbable running suture. A bladder catheter and vaginal packing are placed temporarily and removed in the recovery room when the patient is awake. A voiding trial can be immediately performed.

MiniArc (Figures 12.4A and B) and Solyx Single-Incision Sling

1. Placement of both the MiniArc and Solyx mini slings proceeds by the same initial steps as outlined previously (steps 1-4). The direction of dissection is aimed at a 45-degree angle to the midline, toward the location of the insertion of the adductor longus tendon on the pubic ramus.
2. *Preparation of the sling:* The sling is prepared by inserting the tip of the delivery device or needle into the self-affixing end of the mesh apparatus, ensuring that the mesh is orientated on the outside of bend of the delivery needle.
3. *Insertion of sling:* To place the MiniArc or Solyx mini slings, the tip of the delivery needle with mesh assembly attached is inserted into the previously dissected vaginal space and aimed along a path 45 degrees from the midline. Placement should be immediately posterior to the ischiopubic ramus; the needle can be "walked off" the posterior aspect of the bone as described previously, maintaining a close proximity to the posterior surface of the bone.

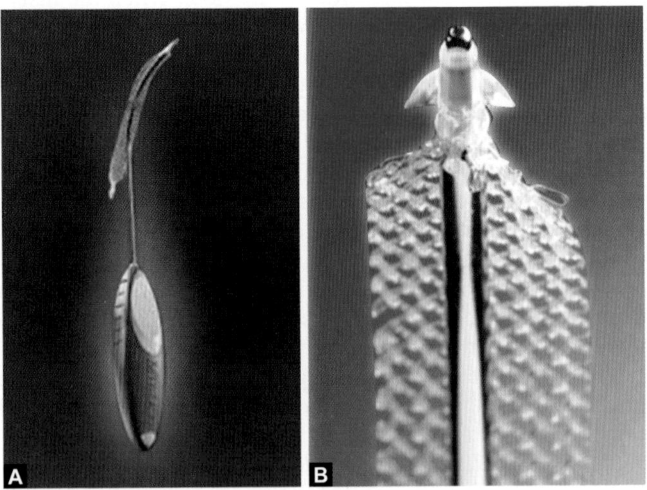

Figures 12.4A and B: MiniArc sling loaded on inserter

The tip should be advanced until the midline marking on the mesh is situated under the middle of the urethra. The needle is removed from the mesh, attached to the other end of the mesh device, and inserted on the contralateral side in a similar manner, ensuring the mesh lies flat under the urethra, until the proper degree of desired tension is achieved. The delivery device is disengaged and removed. The MiniArc single-incision sling can be arranged with a delivery/inserter needle to facilitate reconnecting the needle tip into the self-affixing tip of the mesh device. This arrangement allows for the mesh to be inserted further, if more tension is desired. The redocking procedure entails threading a 2-0 polypropylene suture through the tip of the mesh assembly and then through the tip of the delivery device, knotting one end. This end of the mesh is placed first, in the usual fashion, and then the delivery needle is removed, leaving the suture in place. The opposite side is also placed as described previously. If further tensioning is warranted, the free end of the suture is reinserted into the end of the delivery needle, and the needle is advanced along the suture, sliding into the tip of the mesh device. Once docked, the entire mesh device can be advanced further into the patient.

4. *Cystoscopy:* Cystoscopy may be performed to evaluate for bladder injury.
5. *Vaginal closure:* The vaginal incision is closed in the same way as described previously.

AJUST Adjustable Single-Incision Sling

1. Placement of the AJUST proceeds by the same initial steps (Steps 1-4) as previously outlined.
2. After appropriate dissection is completed, the fixed anchor is pushed into the tissue until it is slightly beyond the ischiopubic ramus. The handle is pivoted toward the obturator internus muscle and membrane. It should be ensured that the midline indicator is at or slightly past the midurethra in the direction of insertion.
3. The fixed anchor is released by pushing the anchor release lever forward, and the introducer is removed. Gentle traction is applied to the suburethral sling to confirm proper fixation.
4. The adjustable anchor is loaded into the introducer and secured by retracting the anchor release lever. Step 1 through Step 3 are repeated on the contralateral side.
5. The adjustable anchor is stabilized at its insertion point while gently pulling on the adjustment tab, and the sling is adjusted. To loosen the

sling, gentle counter traction is applied to the suburethral sling on the adjustable side of the sling implant.
6. When proper sling placement is achieved, the flexible stylet is inserted into the adjusting tab opening, and the slide lock is pushed into place up to the adjustable anchor.
7. The stylet is withdrawn, the excess adjustment mesh lateral to the urethra at the level of the anterior sulcus is trimmed, and the vaginal incision is closed.

Complications and Surgical Tips

Complications that can occur are similar to the complications previously discussed in regard to retropubic and transobturator MUS. These include bladder injury or perforation, bleeding, vaginal mesh extrusion, urinary tract mesh erosion, voiding dysfunction, and urinary retention. Viscous organ damage and major vascular injury still may occur but in theory should be much less common because the needle/trocar trajectory through the retropubic or obturator space is significantly more truncated by design of the mini sling.

Bladder perforation may occur at the time of sling insertion; the self-affixing points of the MiniArc single-incision sling and Solyx SIS may make removal and reinsertion of the device difficult because these slings are not designed to be removed. Removal of the TVT-Secur is accomplished by pulling out the inserted arm that is still attached to the mesh. Removal of the Sling may be facilitated by setting up the redocking procedure with a suture. If bladder perforation occurs and is discovered on cystoscopy, the sling should be immediately removed. A secondary insertion should not be attempted at that operative time. Cystoscopy should be routinely performed at the time of placement of the sling.

Because of the shorter length of inserted mesh, more tension is placed on the mini sling at the time of insertion than is placed on the other types of MUS. The implanted sling should be in close opposition to the urethra with no laxity in the material. The surgeon should use a clamp or long artery forceps to determine that there is no redundancy in the sling material.

Outcomes

Barber et al (2012), De Ridder et al (2010) and Neuman et al (2011) showed similar cure rates when compared to retropubic or transobturator MUS, whereas Wang et al (2011) and Hinoul et al (2011) showed higher long-term cure rates for retropubic or transobturator MUS.

The study by Abdel-Fattah et al (2011) found that single-incision slings were associated with shorter operative times and lower pain scores immediately postoperatively.

Conclusion

At the present time, the future of single-incision slings is questionable because the FDA has required the manufacturers of these kits to pursue further studies to evaluate efficacy and safety. If the data eventually demonstrate acceptable long-term durability and safety, increased popularity is likely owing to the minimal invasiveness of these procedures.

Bibliography

1. Abdel Fatah M, Ford JA Lim CP, Madhuvrata P. Single incision minisling versus standard midurethral sling in management of stress urinary incontinence in females. A meta-analysis of effectiveness and complications. Eur Urol. 2011;60:468-80.
2. Annett Gauruder-Burmester, Gralf Popken. The MiniArc® sling system in the treatment of female stress urinary incontinence. Int Braz J Urol. Rio de Janeiro 2009,35(1):3.
3. Barber MD, Weidner AC, Sokol AI, et al. Foundation of female health awareness Research network. Single incision minisling compared to tension free vaginal tape for the treatment of stress urinary incontinence a randomized controlled trial. Obstet Gynecol. 2012;119:328-37.
4. Castillo-Pinto E, Sasson A, Pons J Comparison of retropubic and transobturator tension-free vaginal implants for the treatment of stress urinary incontinence. Int J Gynecol Obstet. 2010;110:23-6.
5. Chen YH, Wang YJ, Li FP, Wang Q. Efficacy and postoperative complication of tension-free vaginal tape-Secur for female stress urinary incontinence. Chin Med J (Engl). 2011;124(9):1296-1309.
6. Deole N, Kaufmann A, Arunkalaivanan A Evaluation of safety and efficacy in single-incision midurethral short tape procedure (MiniArc™ tape) for stress urinary incontinence under local anesthesia. Int Urogynecol J. 2010;22:335-9.
7. De RD, Berkers J, Deprest J, Verguts J, Ost D, Hamid D, Aa F. Single incision mini-sling versus a transobutaror sling: a comparative study on MiniArc and Monarc slings. Int Urogynecol J Pelvic Floor Dysfunct. 2010;21(7):773-8.
8. Hinoul P, Vervest HA, Den Boon J, et al. A randomized, controlled trial comparing an innovative single incision sling with an established

transobturator sling to treat female stress urinary incontinence. J Urol. 2011;185:1356-62.

9. Kennelly MJ, Moore R, Nguyen JN, Lukban JC, Siegel S. Prospective evaluation of a single incision sling for stress urinary incontinence. J Urol. 2010;184(2):604-9.
10. Moore RD, Mitchell GK, Miklos JR. Single-center retrospective study of the technique, safety, and 12-month efficacy of the MiniArc™ single-incision sling: a new minimally invasive procedure for treatment of female SUI. Surg Technol Int. 2009;18:175-81.
11. Neuman M, Sosnovski V, Kais M, Ophir E, Bornstein J. Transobturator vs single-incision suburethral mini-slings for treatment of female stress urinary incontinence: early postoperative pain and 3-year follow-up. J Minim Invasive Gynecol. 2011;18(6):769-73.

CHAPTER

13

Choice of Surgery for Stress Urinary Incontinence

Sanjay Sinha, Rooma Sinha

Preoperative Caveats

Conservative therapy seldom cures women with bothersome stress urinary incontinence although varying degrees of improvement may be noted. An initial trial of conservative therapies is appropriate especially for women with a low degree of bother. Prior to surgery, it is critically important that the surgeon demonstrate stress urinary incontinence. This can be achieved by a stress test in the outpatient room or by urodynamics evaluation. Failure to demonstrate stress incontinence prior to surgery can lead to inappropriate surgery. One must also exclude a large residual urine volume. While it is possible for women with stress incontinence to show some residual urine, large volumes must prompt the search for an alternate primary diagnosis. All too often, management of the other pathology will render stress incontinence surgery superfluous.

The presence and severity of urgency and frequency should be recorded carefully. Overactive bladder (OAB) symptoms or urodynamic detrusor overactivity is not a contraindication to stress incontinence surgery but outcomes may be poorer. This is especially true for women who have high-pressure detrusor overactivity. Such women must be counseled carefully preoperatively. Pelvic floor assessment should lead to a comprehensive management plan that addresses other concerns such as symptomatic pelvic organ prolapse simultaneously. Women with overt vaginal or urinary infection must undergo treatment before surgery and diabetics should have good glycemic control.

Surgical Options

The various surgical options for stress urinary incontinence can be classified into one of the following groups—retropubic surgery, slings, periurethral injection and the artificial sphincter. One can rapidly narrow down the choice of surgical therapy to a few procedures by an evaluation of the relevant literature. Needle suspension and anterior repair should no longer be offered as surgical treatment for stress incontinence although the latter remains an important surgery for pelvic organ prolapse.

Of the retropubic surgeries, the Burch colposuspension is the standard procedure with durable outcomes and a low complication rate. The Marshall-Marchetti-Krantz procedure is no longer recommended by the International Consultation on Incontinence.[1] While short-term results are comparable, long-term results are inferior to the Burch colposuspension and there is a higher complication rate associated with the procedure. The laparoscopic Burch operation shows an equivalent outcome compared to the standard Burch in recent studies.[2] However, with the advent of synthetic tapes that possibly offer a better outcome with even lesser morbidity, the future of this operation is uncertain.

Of the sling procedures, the autologous fascial sling and the synthetic sling have consistent good outcomes but the allogenic material (such as cadaveric fascia lata) and xenograft material (such as bovine dermis) have dismal medium term outcomes and should probably not be offered. The retropubic tension free vaginal tape as well as the transobturator tapes have been studied in great detail in literature and appear to offer durable outcomes.[3] More recently, there has been interest in single incision mini-slings that are placed in the general direction typically taken by the classical retropubic or transobturator tapes. The intention behind further making the tapes less invasive has been a further reduction in complications, pain and anesthesia requirement. However, good quality medium and long-term data about their efficacy is currently lacking. The available evidence suggests that they are associated with less immediate pain but are also more likely to fail in the medium term.[2]

Results with periurethral injections are unpredictable and the medium term cure rates are dismal.[4] Hence, this procedure would not be a usual first choice for stress incontinence. Artificial sphincter surgery is overkill for the usual patient with stress incontinence and carries a high rate of erosion, revision and failure in women with multiple failed surgeries with scarred and poor quality vaginal tissue.[1] Currently, transurethral injections of stem cells, myoblasts and fibroblast injections are under evaluation.

The sections below will assess the evidence in given specific situations in greater detail. Most of the following discussion will focus on the retropubic midurethral sling, the transobturator midurethral sling, the autologous fascial sling and the Burch colposuspension.

Uncomplicated Stress Urinary Incontinence ("Classical" Presentation)

Women with uncomplicated "classical" presentation have stress incontinence symptoms without any associated voiding difficulty or urgency. They have low residual urine volume and show leakage of urine during an outpatient stress test precisely at the time of the cough. They do not have any other major pelvic floor abnormality and have good quality vaginal tissues.

The outcome of various commonly performed surgical procedures has been evaluated in detail. Ogah et al compared Burch colposuspension with synthetic tapes and showed that there was no difference in short term or medium term outcome in efficacy in a detailed Cochrane review.[5] As would be expected, hospital stay and operating time was longer with the Burch colposuspension. Urinary tract injury was more common with tapes while postoperative pelvic organ prolapse, chiefly posterior compartment due to alteration in the vaginal axis, was more likely with the Burch colposuspension. In a landmark study, Albo et al compared the Burch colposuspension with the autologous sling and found that slings were more effective in terms of stress incontinence-specific success, overall success and patient satisfaction.[6] However, voiding dysfunction occurred in 14 percent of the patients who underwent sling as compared with 2 percent undergoing the Burch. In fact, all the take-downs of the original procedure happened in the sling group.

Rehman et al compared tapes with the autologous sling in a Cochrane review recently and found that they were equivalent in efficacy.[7] The tapes were however, associated with a lower incidence of *de novo* detrusor overactivity and took considerably lesser time to perform. Richter et al compared retropubic tension-free vaginal tape (TVT) with the transobturator tapes (TOTs) in a landmark rigorously conducted trial and found them to be equivalent in efficacy at 12 months. There does not appear to be any major difference in efficacy between the inside-out and outside-in approaches. The retropubic approach is associated with a higher incidence of voiding dysfunction and bladder injury while the transobturator approach is associated with a higher chance of groin pain or numbness and vaginal exposure of the tape. At least some part of the latter is probably due to perforation at the time of the surgery that could not be identified.

In patients with uncomplicated stress urinary incontinence (SUI), based on the above evidence a synthetic tape surgery seems the most logical choice. The type of tape is probably more a matter of surgeon preference. One must recognize that long-term data of 10 years and above, is not yet available for the TOTs.

Mixed Urinary Incontinence

The term "mixed" has been used variously by different publications and this lack of homogeneity is a major stumbling block in the interpretation of literature.[8] The term has been used to include those women who have stress incontinence along with urgency, urgency incontinence, detrusor overactivity or detrusor overactivity incontinence. It is quite obvious that each of these presentations has a different clinical implication.

About 10 percent of women in the UITN trials had detrusor overactivity.[9] The outcome in these women was similar to the rest of the group. However, high-pressure detrusor overactivity of pressure >25 cm H_2O is associated with a poorer outcome.[10] Those who have significant urgency symptoms are more likely to be unsatisfied after their surgery. One should probably choose to treat the urgency first in those women with predominant urgency symptoms. In those women who have predominant stress incontinence symptoms, one could go ahead with SUI surgery after a detailed discussion on the need for postoperative anticholinergic therapy. Resolution rates for stress incontinence are no different in this group. In fact, in some women, stress incontinence may present as urgency. Such women may find that surgery resolves their urgency symptoms. Overall, 24 to 90 percent of women will show resolution of OAB symptoms following SUI surgery.[11,12]

Intrinsic Sphincter Deficiency

Contemporary research shows that most women with stress incontinence will have hypermobility as well as intrinsic sphincter deficiency (ISD) and that patients present a spectrum from isolated ISD to significant hypermobility. Hence, the erstwhile practice of segregating the discussion on the basis of hypermobility or ISD is probably inappropriate. Traditionally, ISD has been defined by urodynamics as an abdominal leak point pressure of <60 cm H_2O or maximal urethral closure pressure of <20 cm H_2O or both.[11,12]

Historically, autologous slings have been the most commonly-performed surgery for patients with ISD and in this group they give cure rates of upwards of 80 percent. However, good quality data is not available for such patients. In a small series, Rezapour et al found TVT to deliver success rates approaching patients without ISD (74% cure and 12% improved).[13] However, five of the eight patients with a fixed, immobile urethra failed. In the rigorously perfomed TOMUS trial, the outcome for both retropubic TVT and transobturator tape was noted to be equivalent. However, such patients were twice as likely to have a failure.

There is data to suggest that those women who have fixed immobile urethra may behave differently from those with hypermobility along with a component of ISD. For such women, an autologous sling still remains the best option. One needs to discuss the possible need for intermittent self-catheterization preoperatively since the sling may need to be kept considerably snug as compared to the usual. One might also consider periurethral injections in this group provided the patient understands that the results are unpredictable and multiple sittings might be required.[11,12]

Recurrent Stress Urinary Incontinence

The long-term failure rate of midurethral slings, the most commonly performed surgery, is about 5 to 20 percent.[11,12] Urethral incompetence is more likely in women with recurrent stress incontinence and some women may have a fixed urethra. Commonly performed surgeries for recurrent stress incontinence include a repeat midurethral sling, autologous pubovaginal sling and occasionally, injection of periurethral bulking agents.

A retrospective study from Australia compared 77 patients undergoing redo surgery with over 1075 patients undergoing a primary procedure.[14] The authors noted that the conventional retropubic tape performed better as compared to a transobturator tape irrespective of whether the initial procedure was a TVT or a transobturator tape. However, the outcome of repeat surgery was poorer as compared with primary procedures (62% versus 86%). Periurethral bulking agents carry a low success of about 35 percent. The autologous pubovaginal sling is an important salvage procedure for patients with recurrent incontinence. Second and third repeat colposuspension surgery carries a low success rate (81% for first repeat, 25% for second and 0% for third redo surgery).[15] Patients with recurrent incontinence must have urodynamics evaluation prior to surgical re-treatment.

Obese Women

Obese women are more likely to present with severe symptoms. They are also more likely to report mixed incontinence. Diary records usually show a higher incontinence episode frequency for such women and they may have a lesser degree of hypermobility. Failure rates for surgery seem to be higher for obese women although good quality data is lacking. Women who are morbidly obese (BMI >35) are specifically at a greater risk of failure.[1] There is evidence to show that an autologous sling is effective in morbidly obese women. In a small series, all 12 women who underwent the procedure became continent.[16] A meta-analysis in which 453 obese women were compared to 1186 nonobese women showed a higher risk of failure of midurethral slings in the obese.[17]

A midurethral sling is a good minimally invasive option in obese women. Patients must be counseled that their outcomes are likely to be inferior irrespective of the procedure chosen. This is especially likely to be true for women who are morbidly obese.

Women Undergoing Concomitant Surgery

Pelvic organ prolapse is a common finding in women undergoing stress incontinence surgery. While a comprehensive pelvic floor management is recommended one needs to guard against an over-zealous approach. To consider repair of pelvic organ prolapse, the woman should have a symptomatic prolapse. The only symptom that consistently correlates with prolapse seems to be a feeling of bulge. Other symptoms such as difficulty in voiding and splinting while voiding urine or defecating, do not show a consistent association with prolapse and may not resolve following surgery for prolapse. In women with symptomatic pelvic organ prolapse, one can safely perform concomitant prolapse surgery without impacting the outcome of stress incontinence surgery.[1] If a midurethral sling is being performed, it is advisable to use a separate incision for the two procedures.

A related issue is the need for stress incontinence surgery in women undergoing prolapse repair. Strictly speaking, this is a discussion for an essay on prolapse rather than stress incontinence. One can summarize the decision-making matrix in the following way. Women who have pelvic organ prolapse but no clinical or occult stress incontinence should probably not be offered a (truly) prophylactic incontinence surgery. Women who have symptomatic stress incontinence (overt) along with prolapse should be offered both surgeries simultaneously. Women who have demonstrable stress incontinence only when their prolapse is reduced and who have no symptoms (occult), should be offered the options of one-step or sequential therapy with a detailed discussion. They must be informed that they have a 10 to 20 percent likelihood of developing symptomatic stress incontinence after prolapse surgery alone. This likelihood is strongly impacted by the degree of prolapse in the cohort. In a study comparing women who underwent abdominal sacrocolpopexy with or without a prophylactic Burch, postoperative stress incontinence was noted in 24 percent in those who underwent the Burch versus 44 percent in the control group and the trial was stopped early.[18] However, if they undergo a simultaneous stress incontinence surgery there is a small chance that they will have new onset voiding dysfunction, which they never had prior to intervention. Also, prophylactic surgery is not uniformly effective.

In women undergoing concomitant pelvic surgery, most often hysterectomy, stress incontinence surgery can be performed with equivalent success rates and without a significant increase in the complication rate. If an open surgery is being contemplated, one may consider a Burch colposuspension. However, one could just as well place a midurethral sling in these women through a vaginal approach.

Elderly Women

Most studies in literature consider women above the age of 70 years as elderly. Elderly women differ from their younger counterparts in several ways. They are more likely to present with mixed incontinence, more likely to have voiding dysfunction due to a weak detrusor muscle and hence, elevated residuals. Preoperative detrusor overactivity is noted in one-fourth of women as compared to about 10 percent of the younger cohort. The quality of vaginal tissues is more likely to be poor with a possible impact on vaginal exposure of synthetic tapes. However, most series suggest that vaginal exposure is not significantly more common in the elderly.[1]

Elderly women are also more likely to suffer age-associated cardiovascular, thromboembolic and pulmonary complications and an action plan to prevent, recognize and treat these problems is mandatory.[1]

Elderly women are more likely to develop postoperative *de novo* urgency and voiding dysfunction. There may be a case for the placement of a transobturator tape in such women due to the less obstructive trajectory of the tape.

References

1. Smith ARB, Dmochowski R, Hilton P, et al. Surgery for urinary incontinence in women. In: Abrams P, Cardozo L, Khoury S, Wein A (Eds) Incontinence, 4th edn. Health Publications, Plymouth. 2009. pp. 1191-272.
2. Lucas, MG, Bosch, JLHR, Cruz, F, et al. Guidelines on urinary incontinence. European Association of Urology 2012. Accessed from www.uroweb.org
3. Richter HE, Albo ME, Zyczynski HM, et al. Retropubic versus transobturator midurethral slings for stress incontinence. N Engl J Med. 2010;362:2066-76.
4. Chrouser KL, Fick F, Goel A, Itano NB, Sweat SD, Lightner DJ. Carbon coated zirconium beads in beta-glucan gel and bovine glutaraldehyde cross-linked collagen injections for intrinsic sphincter deficiency: continence and satisfaction after extended follow-up. J Urol. 2004;171:1152-5.

5. Ogah J, Cody JD, Rogerson L. Minimally invasive synthetic suburethral sling operations for stress urinary incontinence in women. Cochrane Database Syst Rev. 2009;(4):CD006375.
6. Albo ME, Richter HE, Brubaker L, et al. Burch colposuspension versus fascial sling to reduce urinary stress incontinence. N Engl J Med. 2007; 356: 2143-55.
7. Rehman H, Bezerra CC, Bruschini H, et al. Traditional suburethral sling operations for urinary incontinence in women. Cochrane Database Syst Rev. 2011;19(1): CD001754.
8. Sinha S. Approach to the evaluation and treatment of stress urinary incontinence in women. Apollo Med. 2013:10;67-73.
9. Nager C, Albo M, FitzGerald MP, et al. Reference urodynamic values for stress incontinent women. Neurourol Urodyn. 2007;26:333-40.
10. Hosker G, Rosier P, Gajewski J, et al. Dynamic Testing. Incontinence: 4th International Consultation on Incontinence. United Kingdom: Health Publications. 2009. p. 413.
11. Ridgeway B, Barber MD. Midurethral slings for stress urinary incontinence: a urogynecology perspective. Urol Clin North Am. 2012;39:289-97.
12. Lee E, Nitti VW, Brucker BM. Midurethral slings for all stress incontinence: a urology perspective. Urol Clin North Am. 2012;39:299-310.
13. Rezapour M, Falconer C, Ulmsten U. Tension-free vaginal tape (TVT) in stress incontinent women with intrinsic sphincter deficiency (ISD)—a long-term follow-up. Int Urogynecol J Pelvic Floor Dysfunct. 2001;12 Suppl 2:S12-14.
14. Stav K, Dwyer PL, Rosamilia A, et al. Repeat synthetic midurethral sling procedure for women with recurrent stress urinary incontinence. J Urol. 2010;183:241-6.
15. Amaye-Obu FA, Drutz HP. Surgical management of recurrent stress urinary incontinence: A 12-year experience. Am J Obstet Gynecol. 1999; 181:1296-307.
16. Cummings JM, Boullier JA and Parra RO. Surgical correction of stress incontinence in morbidly obese women. J Urol. 1998;160:754-5.
17. Greer WJ, Richter HE, Bartolucci AA and Burgio KL. Obesity and pelvic floor disorders: A systematic review. Obstet Gynecol. 2008;112;341-9.
18. Brubaker L, Cundiff GW, Fine P, et al. Abdominal sacrocolpopexy with Burch colposuspension to reduce urinary stress incontinence. N Engl J Med. 2006;354:1557-66.

CHAPTER

14

Long-term Outcomes of Stress Urinary Incontinence Sling Surgery

A Tamilselvi, Jay Iyer, Ajay Rane

Introduction

Stress urinary incontinence (SUI) is a common condition in women that significantly compromises the quality of life of the sufferers. The terminology genuine stress incontinence has been substituted by stress urinary incontinence. While SUI is a clinical diagnosis, the occurrence of involuntary leakage of urine during urodynamic testing associated with an increased abdominal pressure, in the absence of detrusor contraction is defined as urodynamic stress incontinence.[1]

Epidemiology

The prevalence of urinary incontinence increases with age. Among young adults and middle aged, it is reported in 25 percent of women and in those aged 40 and over the mean prevalence is 34 percent.[2] In geographical terms, Australia is the driest continent on earth; regrettably the same cannot be said of its inhabitants. Studies show that 5 to 6 percent of adult Australians have regular or severe urinary incontinence, prevalence remarkably similar to that reported from other basically Caucasian populations.[3,4]

Data regarding prevalence in Australia have been available since a study performed in Sydney in 1983.[5] No systematic study of general prevalence has been conducted since that time. However, the longitudinal Women's Health Australia study, involving over 40,000 women has provided new data on prevalence in women and may yield further data on the incidence of incontinence over the next 10 to 20 years as the cohorts age.[6,7]

Apart from increasing age, pregnancy and childbirth, White and Hispanic race, pelvic surgery, smoking and obesity are some of the other risk factors implicated in the etiology of SUI. Lifestyle interventions such as weight reduction and pelvic floor exercises remain the primary modality of treatment in women with SUI. If conservative management is unsuccessful, surgical treatment becomes the next option. There is a wide array of surgical techniques available sometimes making the choice of procedure confusing. This chapter aims to outline the long-term outcome and complications of the different surgical techniques in the management of SUI.

Surgical Management

The objective of the urinary anti-incontinence surgery is to restore continence without creating outlet obstruction. Several different surgical options exist for the treatment of urinary stress incontinence and most of these procedures, either aim to stabilize the urethral descent and/or enhance the urethral sphincter function. Different surgical procedures have evolved with renewed understanding of the pathophysiology of SUI. The integral theory of pelvic organ support and midurethral supports in particular, credited to the work by Professor Ulmsten and Professor Petros led to the development of midurethral slings which continue to be the mainstay in the surgical management of SUI.

Anterior Repair with Kelly Plication

Historically, this repair technique employed by gynecologists for a long time was based on the anatomic theory of Bonney. He postulated that SUI occurs due to laxity of the distal part of the pubocervical muscle sheet.[8] This was further endorsed by Kelly who attributed SUI to funneling of the bladder neck secondary to the loss of anterior vaginal wall support. Kelly and Dumm first described the traditional Kelly plication and anterior vaginal repair in 1914.[9] The procedure was performed for nearly 50 odd years for patients with SUI with various modifications of the Kelly technique. However, studies indicate that the operation has a varied success rate of 30 to 70 percent and the success rate decreases with time. Due to the dismal long-term success rates, Kelly plication with anterior colporrhaphy is no longer recommended for the correction of stress urinary incontinence.

Bladder Neck Suspension Procedures

Needle suspension and retropubic bladder neck suspension procedures were based on the pressure transmission theory by Enhorning in 1961.[10] In women who were continent of urine, he showed that the urethral pressure exceeded the vesical pressure both at rest and during increase in intra-abdominal pressure. He hypothesized that this was due to transmission of intra-abdominal pressure equally to the bladder and the proximal urethra above the pelvic floor. In patients with SUI, descent of the proximal urethra below the pelvic floor leads to decrease in urethral pressure and consequent incontinence.

Marshall-Marchetti-Krantz (Retropubic Urethropexy)—MMK Procedure

Marshall-Marchetti-Krantz first described the procedure in 1949. The sutures are placed on either side of the urethra through the pubocervical fascia via abdominal approach. Sutures are then fixed to the periosteum of superior pubic rami, thus elevating bladder neck. Early subjective cure rates were reported to be around 75 to 89 percent but the objective cure rates were lower. The main short to medium term complication, however, was osteitis pubis (2.5–7%) and occasionally leading to osteomyelitis.[11] However, the major long-term complication is severe voiding dysfunction with some patients being compelled to actually stand to void! The procedure became obsolete due to low long-term cure rates and significant procedure related complications and is no longer recommended.

Burch Colposuspension

Burch colposuspension technique involves entry into retropubic space via extraperitoneal approach. The paravaginal tissues at the level of bladder neck are elevated to the ipsilateral ileopectineal ligament (Cooper's) with two or three sutures. The aim is to restore the urethrovesical junction to the retropubic position above pelvic floor. The objective cure rate is estimated to be around 84 to 90 percent at one year. With long-term follow-up studies, Burch colposuspension has a success rate of 85 percent at 5 years.[12] With its good long-term cure rates, colposuspension has long been considered the 'gold standard' surgery for the treatment of SUI. Since its first description in 1961, the procedure has undergone modifications to minimize the complications while maintaining efficacy.

Major intraoperative complications were bleeding and damage to adjacent structures like bladder, urethra, bowel and vessels. The long-term postoperative complications of Burch colposuspension included voiding dysfunction and detrusor overactivity. *De novo* detrusor overactivity occurred in 10 to 12 percent of women postoperatively and 11 to 20 percent had voiding dysfunction at 3 months follow-up.[13]

Posterior compartment defects and enterocele (7–18%) occurred in the long-term due to transmission of abdominal pressure to posterior vaginal wall following the colposuspension.

Laparoscopic Colposuspension

Laparoscopic colposuspension became popular in the 1990s in keeping with the trend towards less invasive procedures. The success rate at one year was 84 percent with laparoscopic approach compared to 95.6 percent with open procedure. There was a decline in the success rates with long-term follow-up.[14] With the laparoscopic approach the incidence of urinary tract injury is 10 percent.[15] However, in comparison with open procedure, no significant differences were observed for postoperative urgency, voiding dysfunction or *de novo* detrusor overactivity. The laparoscopic group had less intraoperative blood loss and significantly shorter hospital stay. In spite of the low morbidity with laparoscopy, based on the poor long-term results and the increased risk of urinary tract injuries Cochrane review concluded that the performance of laparoscopic approach was poorer compared to open approach. Moreover, with the availability of the effective minimally invasive midurethral slings laparoscopic Burch procedures are only occasionally performed today.

Needle Suspension Procedures

Needle suspension procedures were an attractive option in the 1980s. Pereyra first described such a procedure in the 1959. Stamey, Raz and other authors described variations to this technique. The operations involved suspending sutures either from the vaginal, paravaginal or paraurethral tissues to the anterior abdominal wall with an objective of elevating the bladder neck. Permanent sutures were used for needle suspension procedures. With Pereyra's needle suspension, success rate was 65 percent at 1 year and 43 percent at 5 years.

The incidence of urinary tract injury was 1 to 7 percent with needle suspension. There appeared to be no difference in *de novo* detrusor overactivity or voiding difficulty when compared to colposuspension. However, patients undergoing needle suspensions (Stamey, Raz, and Pereyra) were more likely to experience subjective failure at 1 year than those undergoing colposuspension. The long-term cure rate with needle suspension was also very low for all needle suspension procedures.[16]

The advantages of needle suspension, however are simple, involving short operating time, minimal hospitalization, rapid return to activity and a short learning curve. The disadvantages are formation of vesical stone, rejection of the sutures, infection, vaginal granulation and unacceptably high failure rates. Based on the long-term studies with these procedures, it is unwise to use needle suspension as treatment for SUI and are no longer recommended.

Sling Procedures

Sling procedures are well established in the surgical management of stress urinary incontinence. Traditionally the technique was designed to support and elevate the bladder neck by placing a sling material. Originally described by von Giordano in 1907, the technique involved use of autologous tissue—gracilis muscle flap. Aldridge subsequently used rectus fascia as sling material which became a standardized technique.[17]

Natural slings were commonly autologous fascia either from the thigh or rectus fascia, or allogenic from cadaveric fascia or xenogenic from porcine or bovine dermis. A host of synthetic materials multi-filament and monofilament have been used like mersilene, silastic, polytetrafluoroethylene and polypropylene meshes. With natural slings the rejection rate is lower but they resulted in higher rate of wound infection at the harvested site, hematoma formation and voiding difficulties. Synthetic slings on the other hand are associated with higher risks of graft erosion, rejection and infection mainly with multifilament materials. The pubo-vaginal sling procedures can be done via abdominal approach, vaginal approach or combined abdominal-vaginal approach. The cure rates range from 85 to 90 percent, being comparable to that of colposuspension. The incidence of *de novo* detrusor overactivity is 16.6 percent and voiding difficulty 10 percent.[18]

The good long-term success rates, with the technique avoiding repair using defective tissue and the fact it can treat both urethral hypermobility and ISD shows greater potential for its use. In the traditional sling procedures, autologous fascia were placed under the urethrovesical junction but with the acceptance of the midurethral concept, minimally invasive slings using synthetic sling material have become the sling procedures of choice.

Midurethral Slings

The shift of the sling position from bladder neck to midurethra was the culmination of several theories. The most important of those are the midurethral integral theory hypothesized by Petros and Ulmsten [19] and the Hammock theory suggested by DeLancey.[20] The presence of rich vascular plexus, presence of supportive structures like pubourethral ligaments and urogenital diaphragm and the insertion of pubococcygeus muscle in the vaginal wall at the midurethra supports the midurethral concept.

The functional features that favor the midurethral concept are, detection of maximum closure pressure at midurethra [21] interruption of urinary flow at midurethra on holding, presence of dense innervation at midurethra and detection of highest pressure rise in distal part of urethra on straining.[22] The available anatomical and functional features favoring the midurethral concept, the shift occurred with reference to the site of sling placement from bladder neck to midurethra.

Tension-free vaginal tape (TVT) initially described by Ulmsten was the first of the midurethral slings. With TVT, the polypropylene mesh is placed under the midurethra with minimal tension, via vaginal approach exiting abdominally through the retropubic space. Restoration and reinforcement of supporting structures around the urethra is achieved by facilitating the growth of fibroblast around the sling. In its original description the procedure was done under local anesthesia and sedation, enabling tension to be adjusted according to the degree of incontinence.

Early case series with TVT, quoted objective cure rates of 84 to 100 percent for up to two years. The high success rates have persisted in the long-term studies with 95 percent cure rate at 5 years[23] and 82 percent cure rate at 7 years.[24] The eleven year outcome by the same group also showed a subjective cure rate for SUI to be 77 percent with efficacy lasting for more than 10 years.[25]

The risk of voiding disorders is around 2 percent and that of *de novo* detrusor overactivity is around 5 percent with TVT. The largest randomized controlled trial (RCT) comparing TVT and colposuspension has shown similar objective cure rates for both the procedures, 66 percent with TVT and 57 percent with colposuspension.[26]

The RCT comparing TVT with colposuspension apart from providing the cure rates also brought to light various complications encountered with TVT both in the short-term and long-term.[27] Vascular, bladder and bowel injuries have been the immediate complications reported with TVT procedure. These were thought to be related, at least partly to the blind entry of the needle into the retropubic space. The awareness about these complications had led to the introduction of modified devices, in an attempt to reduce the complication profile of TVT.

The transobturator entry route was proposed and introduced by Delorme with the transobturator tape (TOT). De Lorme designed the transobturator placement of midurethral sling from outside in. Jon De Leval modified the surgical technique by passing the sling from inside out in an attempt to minimize the inadvertent injury to urinary tract.

Available literature reveals that there is no significant difference in the cure rate between the retropubic and transobturator approach. However, there appears to be a significant reduction in the incidence of complications with transobturator route. The results of a multicenter trial with short-term follow-up has shown cure rates of 80.5 percent with no vascular, bowel or nerve injury.[28, 29]

Currently both the retropubic approach and the transobturator approach midurethral sling procedures have been widely accepted in the surgical treatment of SUI and form the primary anti-incontinence procedure. They appear to provide good success rates in the treatment of both urethral hypermobility and intrinsic sphincter deficiency.

The complications related to midurethral slings can be either due to the mesh/graft material or due to the trocar insertion.

The specific issues that need to be addressed while considering the long-term complications of current midurethral slings include, erosion or extrusion, voiding dysfunction and pain:

- *Erosion:* Sling exposure or erosion, as it is more commonly referred to, is the exposure of strands of the mesh either suburethral or less commonly the fornix. The patient may be asymptomatic but not uncommonly the patient complains of unusual vaginal discharge or bleeding or the husband may complain of feeling 'sharp strands'. The treatment is simple and involves excision of the offending strands preferably under anesthesia and fascial repair. With minimal exposures in an atrophic vagina, a topical estrogen cream application allows the vaginal tissues to re-epithelize over the mesh.
- *Voiding dysfunction:* This is a more difficult problem to deal with following a sling surgery. Ideally the presence of any voiding dysfunction should have been assessed preoperatively by urodynamic evaluation. If severe voiding dysfunction occurs within a week of surgery and patient repeatedly fails 'trails of void', the only way to treat this is sling division. Voiding problems that occur a few weeks after the surgery and typically after a normal voiding in the immediate postoperative period, may be treated conservatively with timed voiding. The situation invariably resolves with time. It is good practice to perform a 3D/4D ultrasound scan to note the position of the sling and tension on Valsalva. If the sling is close to the bladder neck, instead of the midurethral location, with voiding problem, the sling may have to be divided. Various techniques of sling division have been described, midline sling excision, segmental sling excision and formal urethrolysis. Resolution of voiding problem with these techniques have been quoted around 65 to 93 percent with low rates of recurrence of SUI of 0 to 19 percent.[30,31]
- *Groin pain:* When a transobturator sling is performed it is important to ensure that the adductor longus tendon is palpated and the sling is placed below the tendon medial to the genitor-crural fold. Postoperative groin pains are not simple to treat and the affected area may need to be injected with steroids and local anesthetic. In recalcitrant cases the sling may need to be dissected and removed to the possible extent.

Periurethral Bulking Agents

Edward McGuire in 1977, identified that in a group of patients with surgical failure of incontinence surgery, the bladder neck was in the normal position but the proximal urethra and bladder neck was open even at rest. The urethral resistance was therefore low, leading to incontinence and the condition came to be described as intrinsic sphincter deficiency. The traditional approaches elevating the bladder neck was, hence of no value in this group of patients. Periurethral bulking agents on the other hand aim to increase the urethral outlet resistance and promote continence.

Periurethral bulking injections historically involved the injection of autologous or synthetic agents under the cystoscopic guidance into or around the incompetent urethra. These periurethral bulking agents enhance the internal seal mechanism and stop the flow of urine by effectively coapting the urethral mucosa and thereby increasing the urethral closure pressure. Initially, autologous fat and polytetrafluoroethylene (PTFE) were used. However, the risk of particle migration and granular formation restricted the usage of PTFE.

Currently silicone is used as bulking agent. It has good short-term cure with 50 to 60 percent of patients showing marked improvement of their symptom with no increased risk of major complications.

Injectables remain a reasonable, minimally invasive alternative to surgical repair, both as a primary treatment and as a secondary procedure for recurrent SUI. Due to their mechanism of action, the success rates are higher in those with good bladder neck support but poor urethral function. The long-term success rates are however low with 40 percent cure rate at four-year follow-up.[32] Reasonable short-term cure rates combined with low morbidity makes these procedures ideal in the elderly, with the understanding that repeat injections may be needed.

Artificial Urinary Sphincter

The artificial urinary sphincter has a minimal role in the management of SUI because of the availability of the several different minimally invasive surgical options with low morbidity. The only technique that closely mimics the active mechanism of natural continence is artificial urinary sphincter.

It offers a success rate of 80 percent, but it is associated with complications like fluid leak, erosion or atrophy at the cuff site, kinked tubing, and infection. Main problems which makes it a last resort in surgical options are failure of device and erosion of the cuff.

Conclusion

The surgeries for SUI have undergone several changes over the years and so have the complication profile with each surgery. It is important while counseling patients, that apart from the success rate the likely risks involved in each procedure should be discussed and documented. It would be ideal to provide a written information to supplement the discussion.

New surgical techniques should not be undertaken by the novice without proper training. With the advent of midurethral slings, knowledge about the anatomy of the retropubic space and the trans-obturator spaces in relevance to the adjacent structures became important. With the advent of midurethral slings knowledge about the anatomy of the retropubic space and the transobturator spaces become important—spaces and landmarks, which were not of much significance to the gynecologists or the urologists until then. This meant not only learning the technique but also understanding the relevant anatomy.

The crucial element in minimizing the complications is proper training. Mentoring by a urogynecologist and performing adequate 'numbers' to overcome the training curve are essential. The learning curve for each individual varies and this should be taken into account while deciding on the numbers needed to learn a surgical technique. We surgeons need to remember that we have a primary responsibility of 'not making the cure worse than the disease'.

References

1. Abrams P, Cardozo L, Fall M, Griffiths D, et al. The Standardisation of Terminology of Lower Urinary Tract Function: report from the Standardisation sub-committee of the International Continence Society. Neurourology and Urodynamics. 2002;21:167-78.
2. Thom D. Variation in estimates of urinary incontinence prevalence in the community: effects of differences in definition, population characteristics, and study type. Journal American Geriatric Society. 1998;46:473-80.
3. Thomas TM, Blannin PK J, Meade TW. Prevalence of urinary incontinence. British Medical Journal. 1980;281(6250):1243-5.
4. Jolleys JV. Reported prevalence of urinary incontinence in women in a general practice. British Medical Journal. 1988;296(6632):1300-2.
5. Abstracts of the proceedings of the Urological Society of Australasia, 37th Annual General Meeting, Melbourne, Australia. British Journal of Urology. 1985;57:91-105.

6. Brown WJ, Byles JE, Dobson AJ, Lee C, Mishra G, Schofield M. Women's Health Australia: recruitment for a national longitudinal cohort study. Women and health. 1998;28(1):23-40.
7. Chiarelli P, Brown W, McElduff P. Leaking urine: prevalence and associated factors in Australian women. Neurourology and Urodynamics. 1999;18(6):567-77.
8. Bonney V. On diurnal incontinence of urine in women. J Obstet Gynaecol Br Emp. 1923;30:358-65.
9. Kelly HA, Dumm WM. Urinary incontinence in women, without manifest injury to the bladder. Surg Gynecol Obstet. 1914;18:444-50.
10. Enhörning G, Miller ER, Hinman F Jr. Urethral closure studied with cineroentgenography and simultaneous bladder-urethra pressure recording. Surg Gynecol Obstet. 1964;118:507-16.
11. Odejinmi F, Cutner A. Alternatives to Burch Colposuspension. The Obstetrician and Gynaecologist. 2001;3(3):113-9.
12. Alcalay M, Monga A, Stanton SL, Burch Colposuspension: a 10-20 years follow-up. BJOG. 1995;102:740-5.
13. Lapitan MC, Cody DJ, Grant AM. Open retropubic colposuspension for urinary incontinence in women. The Cochrane Database of Systematic Reviews 2005, Issue 3. CD002912.
14. Moehrer B, Ellis G, Carey M, Wilson PD. Laparoscopic colposuspension for urinary incontinence in women. The Cochrane Database of Systematic Reviews 2000, Issue 3. CD002239.
15. Meyers DL, Peipert JF, Rosenblatt PL, Ferland RJ, Jackson ND. Patient satisfaction with laparoscopic Burch retropubic urethropexy. Journal of Reproductive Medicine. 2000;45:939-43.
16. O'Sullivan DC, Chilton CP, Munson KW. Should Stamey colposuspension be our primary surgery for stress incontinence? British Journal of Urology.1995;75(4):457-60.
17. Aldridge AH. Transplantation of fascia for relief of urinary stress incontinence. Am J Obstet Gynecol.1942;44:398.
18. Bidmead J, Cardoza L. Sling techniques in the treatment of genuine stress incontinence. BJOG. 2000;107:147-56.
19. Petros PE, Ulmsten UI. An Integral theory of female urinary incontinence: experimental and Clinical Considerations. Acta Obstet Gynecol Scand. 1997;166:(Suppl):3-8.
20. DeLancey JO. Structural support of the urethra as it relates to stress urinary Incontinence: the Hammock Hypothesis. American Journal of Obstet Gynaecol. 1994;170(6):1713-20.
21. Westby M, Amussen M, Ulmsten U. Location of maximum intraurethral pressure related to Urogenital diaphragm in the female studied by simultaneous urethrocystometry and voiding cystourethrography. American Journal of Obstet Gynaecol. 1982;144:408-12.

22. Constantinou CE, Govan DE. Spatial distribution and timing of transmitted and reflexly generated urethral pressures in healthy women. Journal of Urology. 1982;127(5):964-9.
23. Nilsson CG, Kuuva N, Falconer C, Rezapour M, Ulmsten U. Long-term results of the tension-free vaginal tape (TVT) procedure for surgical treatment of female stress urinary incontinence. Int Urogynecol J Pelvic Floor Dysfunct. 2001;12(Suppl 2):S5-8.
24. Nilsson CG, Falconer C, Rezapour M. Seven-year followup of the tension-free vaginal tape procedure for treatment of urinary incontinence. Obstet Gynecol. 2004;104:1259-62.
25. Nilsson CG, Palva K, Rezapaour M, Falconer C. Eleven years prospective follow-up of the tension-free vaginal tape procedure for treatment of stress urinary incontinence. Int Urogynecol J. 2008;19: 1043-7.
26. Ward K, Hilton P. Prospective multicentre randomized trial of tension-free vaginal tape and colposuspension as primary treatment for stress incontinence. BMJ. 2002;325:67-70.
27. Ward K, Hilton P. On behalf of the UK and Ireland TVT Trial Group. Tension-free vaginal tape versus colposuspension for primary urodynamic stress incontinence: 5-year follow up. BJOG. 2008;115: 226-33.
28. Costa P, Griese P, Droopy S, Monneins F, et al. Surgical treatment of female stress urinary incontinence with a transobturator tape (TOT). Uratape: short term results of a prospective multicentric study. European Journal of Urology. 2004;46:102-6.
29. Valentim-Lourenco A, Benoun M, Mascarenhas T, Cruz F, Moniz L. TORP—Comparing the efficacy, execution and early complications of TVT and TVT-O. Intl Urogynaecol J. 2008;19 (Suppl 1):S1-S166.
30. Gomelsky A, Nitti VW, Dmochowski RR. Management of obstructive voiding dysfunction after incontinence surgery: lessons learned. Urology. 2003;62:391-3.
31. Starkman JS, Scarpero H, Dmochowski RR. Methods and results of Urethrolysis. Curr Urol Rep. 2006;7:384-94.
32. Corcos J, Fournier C. Periurethral collagen injection for the treatment of female stress urinary incontinence: 4-year follow-up results. Urology. 1999;54:815-8.

CHAPTER

15

Meshplasty for Correction of Stress Urinary Incontinence: Our Experience

RM Saraogi, Mohit Saraogi, Nishita Parekh

Stress urinary incontinence (SUI) is an involuntary loss of urine through an intact urethra due to an increase in the intravesical pressure above the intraurethral pressure which is objectively demonstrable and causes social and hygienic problems.[1]

Stress incontinence affects 15 to 60 percent of all women. It is a disorder of young as well as old women with more than a quarter of nulliparous, young college athletes experiencing stress incontinence while participating in sports.

Surgery must be individualized for each patient, and must follow standard recommendations for appropriate surgery. The option selected depends on the surgeon's training and expertise in a vaginal or abdominal approach. We have older methods like Kelly's repair and abdominal bladder neck suspension surgeries. With recent advances in medical technology and better understanding of female anatomy and physiology, many innovative surgical methods like sling surgeries, tension-free vaginal tape (TVT), transobturator tape (TOT) and Saraogi's meshplasty are now available for correcting stress incontinence.[2]

Saraogi's meshplasty is based on similar principle as other sling procedures (like TVT, TOT).

If one stands on a hosepipe in the lawn and the floor is rigid enough, the pressure of your foot will stop water leakage. But, if the floor is soft, the tube will still be leaking. Now imagine the hosepipe to be the urethra, the floor of the lawn to be the pelvic floor, the pressure of your foot to be Valsalva's maneuver and water leakage to be SUI **(Figure 15.1)**.

Recent advances in knowledge about the pathophysiology of SUI shows that it is the support at the midurethral level which is weak (and not proximal urethra) resulting into sagging of midurethra. Hence, whenever intra-abdominal pressure rises, e.g. Valsalva's maneuver, the intravesical and proximal urethral pressure becomes more than that in midurethra resulting into dribbling of urine, i.e. SUI.

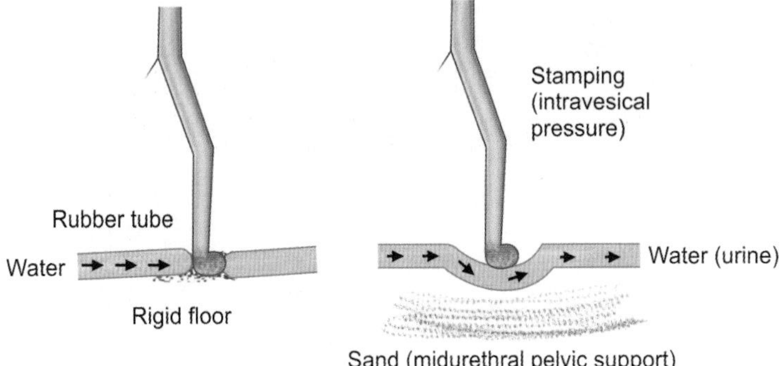

Figure 15.1: Analogy between hosepipe and urethra

It will be irrational to use this already weak and torn fascia to support the urethra. It may give temporary relief but it does not give long-term success, as seen in Kelly's plication sutures. Hence, these supports should be enhanced and re-established using synthetic material, like polypropylene mesh, which will provide permanent solution.

In the technique of Saraogi's meshplasty for SUI correction, the lost fascial support at midurethra is simply re-established by fixing flexible, nonabsorbable, nonreactive polypropylene mesh (Hernia mesh) of size 3 × 2 cm at the midurethral level. The polypropylene mesh[3] provides mechanical support at the place of torn and detached pubovesico-cervical fascia.

The mesh later gets interpenetrated by fibroblasts thus creating a tough underlying fibrous support for the midurethra and causing permanent elevation of midurethra.

Principles of Meshplasty

- The surgery aims at correcting the deficient support at the midurethral level.
- It involves fixation at midurethral level of a flexible yet nonabsorbable, nonreactive polypropylene mesh of approximately 3 cm × 2 cm size with good memory **(Figure 15.2)**.
  - The mesh gets interpenetrated by fibroblasts at a later stage, creating a tough and permanent fibrous support[4] to the midurethra at the site of torn and detached pubocervicovesical vaginal fascia.

A prospective clinical trial was conducted at Corporation Hospital from January 2005 to August 2012 and comprises of 412 cases in which

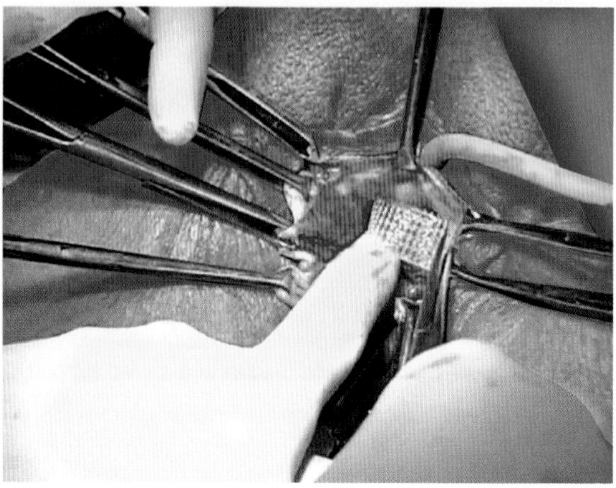

Figure 15.2: Placement of mesh at midurethral level

meshplasty was performed as a choice of surgery for SUI correction. This study was planned to evaluate the feasibility and effectiveness of this procedure in the management of SUI.

Inclusion Criteria

- Any age group and parity
- Clinically demonstrable stress urinary incontinence with or without associated pelvic floor defect
- Positive Marshal and Bonney's test and Q tip test.

Exclusion Criteria

- Urge incontinence
- Urinary tract infections (UTIs)
    - All patients in the inclusion criteria were thoroughly evaluated by detailed history taking, filling an urogynecological symptom based questionnaire and by complete physical and gynecological examination.[5] Any Associated pelvic floor defect was noted.

Stress urinary incontinence was objectively demonstrated by Valsalva's maneuver with full bladder and wherever feasible was confirmed by urodynamic studies.

Investigations

- Complete blood count
- Urine routine and microscopy
- Blood sugar fasting and postprandial

- Wherever needed liver function test, renal function test, electrocardiogram and chest X-ray for anesthesia fitness were performed
- Urodynamic studies whenever feasible.

Treatment

Injection Cefotaxim 1 g intravenously was given to all the patients at the time of induction.

Anesthesia

- Local anesthesia or general anesthesia for only meshplasty
- Spinal anesthesia for meshplasty associated with other pelvic floor repair surgeries.

Surgical Technique

- All surgeries were performed in lithotomy position.
- Saline adrenaline infiltration (1:2,00,000) (when done in GA or SA) or xylocaine—adrenaline (when done under only local anesthesia) was used in all cases **(Figure 15.3A).**
- In patients with dysfunctional uterine bleeding (DUB) or uterine prolapse, vaginal hysterectomy was performed first, followed by dissection of anterior vaginal wall away from underlying pubovesicovaginal fascia (as is being done for anterior colporrhaphy procedure). Dissection was done as laterally as possible **(Figures 15.3B and 15.3C).**
- An indwelling Foley's catheter helped define the midurethra (identified as the middle 1/3rd area between the external urethral meatus and the inflated Foley's bulb lying at bladder neck).
- Then a polypropylene mesh (hernia mesh) of 3 to 4 cm length × 1.5 to 2 cm breadth **(Figures 15.3D and 15.3E)**, was placed at the midurethral level extending from one paraurethral gutter to the other and is fixed with no. 2-0/3-0 vicryl on lateral sides by anchoring its angle with pubocervical fascia along with the vagina at 4 corners **(Figures 15.3F and 15.3G)**. The mesh was fixed in a tension free way so that a small forceps could be easily passed beneath it **(Figure 15.3H)**. After placement of this mesh, anterior colporrhaphy was performed in usual way **(Figure 15.3I)**.
- In patients with only SUI, the mesh was kept (no fixation sutures taken) in the dissected paraurethral spaces on either side at the midurethral level and vagina was closed above it **(Figures 15.4A to D)**. If surgery is done under LA bladder is filled with 200 mL of saline and patient is asked to cough and look for SUI on table itself.

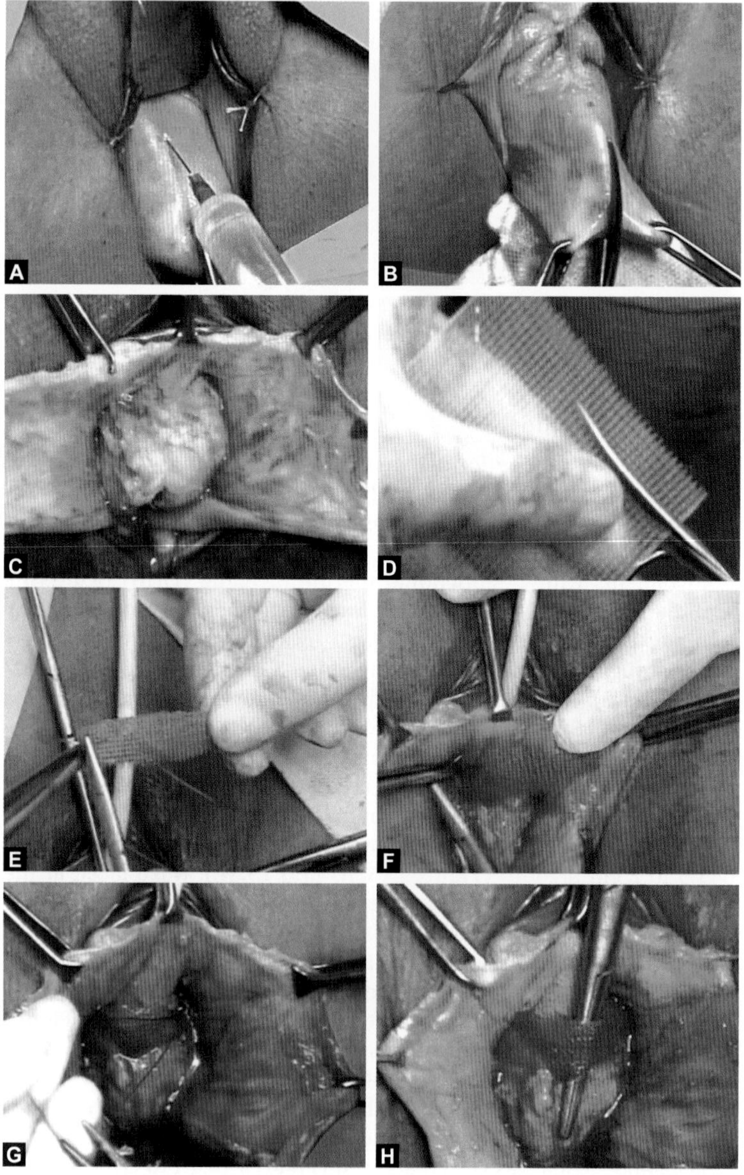

Figures 15.3A to H

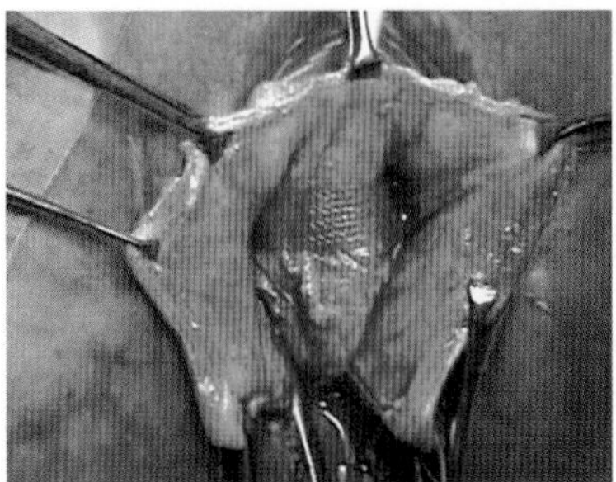

Figure 15.3I

Figures 15.3A to I: Steps of meshplasty during procedure of anterior colporrhaphy

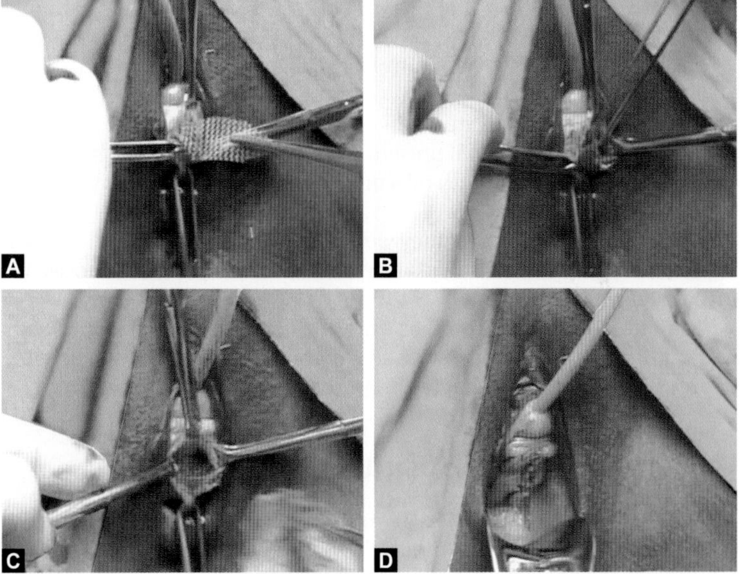

Figures 15.4A to D: Meshplasty in patients with only SUI (no fixation sutures)

Postoperative Care

- Patients were ambulated after 4 hours only if SUI surgery was under LA
- Vaginal pack, if kept (in patients with other associated surgery for prolapse, etc.) was removed the following day
- Antibiotics.

Catheter Removal

- When only meshplasty was performed Foley's catheter is removed on the same evening.
- When associated with anterior colporrhaphy, Foley's catheter was removed on Day 3.
- Residual urine volume was noted
- Any leak on Valsalva maneuver was noted
- Vaginal douche as and when required.

Discharge

At the time of discharge patients were instructed to avoid strenuous physical activity and sexual intercourse for 6 weeks.

Follow-up

- Weekly for 1 month
- During each weekly visit, a mild hydrogen peroxide and betadine vaginal douche was given.
- Pattern of healing was studied.
- Signs of mesh rejection if present were noted.
- Followed by once a month till 6 months and 6 monthly for 2 years and yearly till date.

Further, during each visit they were questioned regarding recurrence of previous symptoms. Also Valsalva maneuver was performed to see for urinary leakage.

The outcomes were noted as cure (absence of urinary complaints and no urinary leakage with Valsalva maneuver) or failure (recurrence of previous symptoms or having demonstrable urinary leakage).

Observation and Results

This prospective clinical trial was conducted at Municipal General Hospital in Mumbai for a period from January 2005 to August 2012, and comprised of 412 cases in which meshplasty was performed as a choice of surgery for SUI correction.

Distribution of Cases in Relation to Parity

The patients with any parity were included in the study population, as shown in **Figure 15.5**.

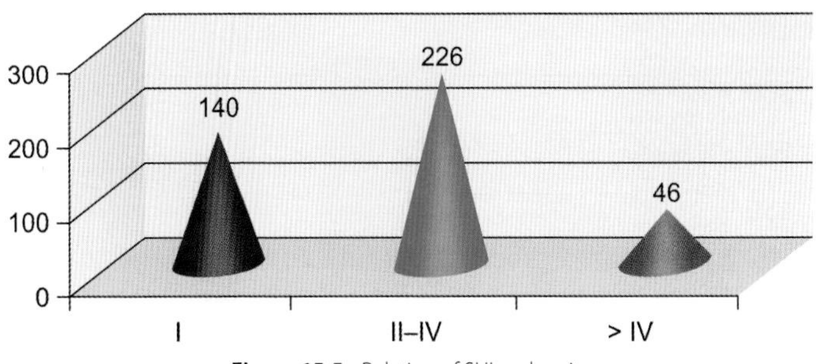

Figure 15.5: Relation of SUI and parity

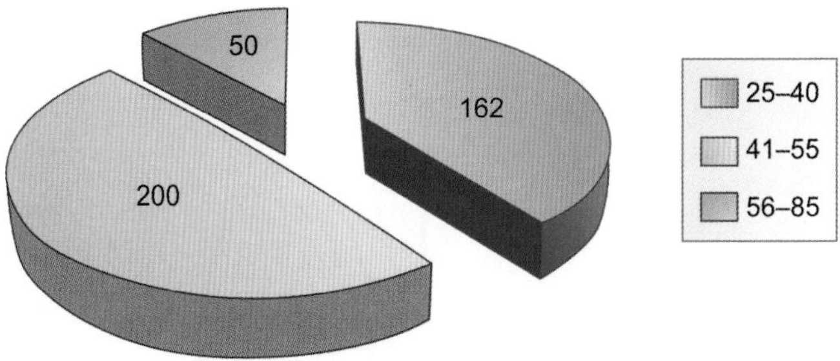

Figure 15.6: SUI in relation with age

Distribution of Cases in Relation to Age

The patients were between age group 28 to 82 years with a total of 412 patients **(Figure 15.6)**.

Age group	Number of patients
25–40	162
41–55	200
56–85	50

Distribution of Cases According to Symptoms

See **Figure 15.7**.

Distribution of Cases in Relation to Type of Anesthesia Used

See **Figure 15.8**.

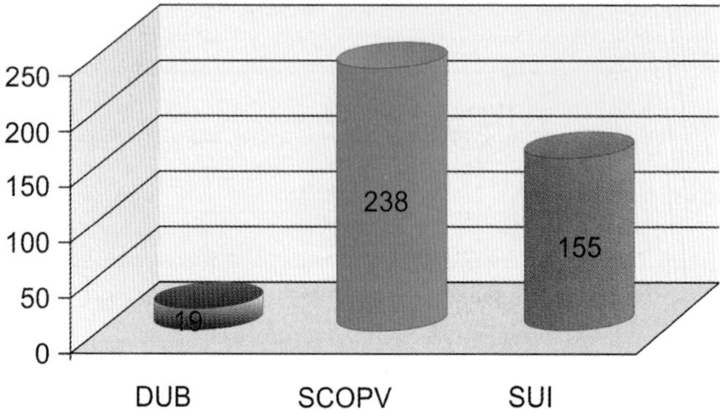

Figure 15.7: SUI and associated symptoms

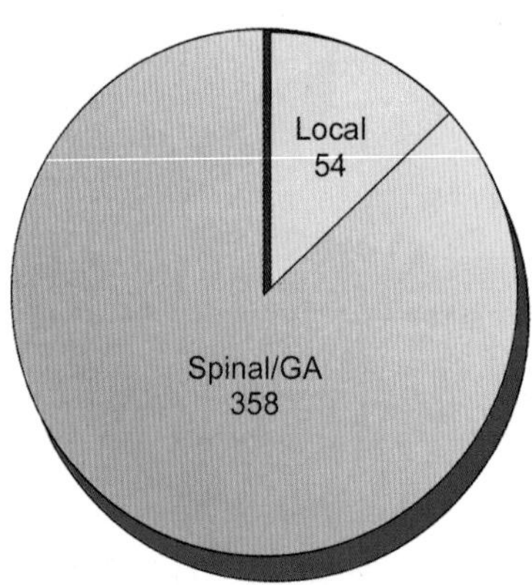

Figure 15.8: SUI surgery and anesthesia given

Distribution of Cases According to Surgical Procedure Performed

In all the patients in the study population, meshplasty was performed as choice of surgery for treatment of SUI. In 155 patients presenting with only SUI as their chief complaint without associated pelvic floor defect, only meshplasty was performed under local anesthesia or GA. In 94 patients, meshplasty was performed along with repair of cystocele and rectocele, i.e. anterior colporrhaphy with posterior colpoperineorrhaphy (A-P repair). In 102 patients with varying degrees of uterine descent, meshplasty was performed along with vaginal hysterectomy and A-P repair. In 24 patients with, procidentia, meshplasty was performed along with vaginal hysterectomy with A-P repair with sacrospinous fixation. In 18 patients with previous hysterectomy and now presented with vault prolapse along with SUI, meshplasty was performed along with vault prolapse repair with sacrospinous fixation. In 19 patients, meshplasty was performed along with vaginal hysterectomy, as shown here:

Surgery	Number of patients
Only meshplasty	155
Cysto-rectocoele repair	94
Vaginal hysterectomy with A-P repair	102
Vaginal hysterectomy with A-P repair with sacrospinous fixation	24
Vault prolapse repair with sacrospinous fixation	18
Vaginal hysterectomy	19

Urodynamic Studies

Preoperative urodynamic study was possible only in 34 cases, while postoperative studies could be done only in 20 cases. Both were showing excellent results.

Complications

Mesh rejection	27 cases	6.55 percent
Recurrence	26 cases	6.31 percent
Retention of urine	4 cases	0.97 percent

Follow-up

- Out of 412 cases, 231 patients are lost to follow-up during different intervals. In the remaining 181 cases, follow-up time varied from 1 month to 7 years.
- The short-term results of meshplasty are also far better than the so called "next wave" of minimally invasive procedures for treatment of SUI like TVT, TOT, and T-SUIT.
- Principle of meshplasty is similar as that of TVT, TOT. However, meshplasty has certain advantages over these procedures like no abdominal incision is required for fixing the tape. The polypropylene mesh can be easily fixed along the para urethral gutters.
- There is no need of intraoperative or postoperative cystoscopy.
- It can be done under local anesthesia.
- It has a short learning curve. It can be performed by a surgeon who can perform anterior colporrhaphy.
- Complications like enterocele, which are common after bladder neck suspension surgeries do not occur following meshplasty.[6]

Summary and Conclusion

- Meshplasty is a very simple and quick procedure.
- Isolated meshplasty procedure required a time period of 10 to 15 minutes only.
- Can be performed under local anesthesia.
- No intraoperative complications, like hemorrhage, injury to bladder, injury to urethra was noted.
- Assistance from other surgical faculties like urology is not required.
- Postoperative complications like febrile morbidity, local and systemic infection was not seen in any of the patients.
- Can be performed along with other ancillary procedures for pelvic floor defect repair.
- Can be performed in patients with medical disorders like hypertension, diabetes, heart disease.
- It is a cost effective procedure in comparison to other procedures used in treatment of SUI.
- Hospital stay of 1 day or maximum 3 days when other ancillary procedures are performed.
- Does not require any special skill or any special surgical instrument.
- Can be performed in remote places where minimum facilities are available with short learning curve.

References

1. Colombo M, Vitobello D, Proiietti F, et al. Randomized comparison of Burch colposuspension vs anterior colporrhaphy in women with SUI and anterior vaginal wall prolapse. BJOG. 2000;107:544-1.
2. Stress urinary incontinence: What, when, why, and then what? J Midlife Health. 2011; 2(2): 57-64.
3. Boukerrou M, Rubod C, Dedet B, Boodhum R, Nayama M, Cosson M. Int Urogynecol J Pelvic Floor Dysfunct. Epub 2007 Sep 14. Tissue resistance of the tension-free procedure: what about healing? 2008;19(3):397-400.
4. Romero Maroto J, Prieto Chaparro L, López López C, Quilez Fenoll JM, Bolufer Nadal S. Prolene mesh sling in the treatment of stress urinary incontinence. Integral treatment of pelvic floor anomalies. Long-term results. Arch Esp Urol. 2002;55(9):1057-74.
5. Nygaard IE, Heit M. Stress urinary incontinence. Obstet Gynecol. 2004;104(3):607-20.
6. Wall LL. Urinary stress incontinence. In: Rock JA, Thompson JD (Eds), Te Linde's operative gynecology, 9th edn. Philadelphia, Lippincott William and Wilkins. 1997:1071.

CHAPTER

16

Voiding Dysfunction and Retention after Stress Urinary Incontinence Surgery

Nishita Parekh, Yugali Warade, Prakash Trivedi

Introduction

The true incidence of voiding dysfunction and iatrogenic obstruction after anti-incontinence surgery is unknown and likely underestimated because of under diagnosis, misdiagnosis, variations in definition and under-reporting. Reported rates of obstruction vary depending on the type of anti-incontinence surgery performed. Urinary obstruction requiring intervention after any anti-incontinence surgery occurs in at least 1 to 2 percent of patients even in the hands of the most experienced surgeon. Voiding dysfunction after surgery for stress urinary incontinence (SUI) can be related to various degrees of obvious outlet obstruction, *de novo* development of detrusor overactivity, or a significant worsening of pre-existing detrusor overactivity.

Historically, textbooks have also discussed the potential for impaired contractility to be a cause in such situations. When patients present with various degrees of voiding dysfunction or symptomatic overactive bladder symptoms, the surgeon must go to great lengths to construct a management plan to address these very distressing symptoms.

Patients with iatrogenic obstruction or voiding dysfunction after surgery for SUI can present with many symptoms. The most obvious signs and symptoms include complete or partial urinary retention, inability to void continuously and the presence of a slow stream with a prolonged voiding time with or without intermittency. Also, many women with milder forms of outlet obstruction complain of having to lean back or even stand up to void. Some women do not have obstructive voiding symptoms and present mainly with the *de novo* development of irritative symptoms of frequency, urgency and urge incontinence. Women may also present with a combination of voiding and storage symptoms. The clinical challenge is to determine whether these symptoms can be directly correlated to the outlet obstruction secondary to either sling placement being too tight or overzealous tightening of suspension sutures.

Transient voiding dysfunction and retention can occur frequently and to a certain degree are expected to occur after certain types of anti-incontinence surgery. It is common for a patient to have retention for days to weeks after a biologic pubovaginal sling or certain suspension procedures. Patients with synthetic sling procedures done in isolation should void immediately postoperatively or shortly thereafter in most cases.

When a surgical intervention for iatrogenic voiding dysfunction is believed to be necessary, controversy exists regarding the timing and techniques for these procedures. Preoperative cystourethroscopy should always be performed because the surgeon needs to ensure there is no sling material or sutures within the urethra or the bladder. Also, depending on the clinical situation, urodynamic studies may be helpful in documenting iatrogenic outlet obstruction as the cause for the patient's symptoms.

Traditionally, evaluation has been delayed for at least 3 months after surgery; this was based on literature following pubovaginal slings, colposuspension, or needle suspension where recurrent SUI after intervention was minimized by waiting at least 90 days. This waiting period that has been advocated for these traditional procedures has largely been abandoned for retropubic, transobturator and single-incision synthetic midurethral sling procedures. Because of immobility of mesh and tremendous in growth of fibroblastic tissue by 2 weeks postoperatively, patients with retention or severe symptoms are unlikely to improve much beyond this time period.

After retropubic and transobturator tape procedures, milder forms of temporary voiding dysfunction have been reported to resolve in 25 to 66 percent of patients in 1 to 2 weeks and 66 to 100 percent of patients by 6 weeks.

Based on these data and our experience, waiting beyond 6 weeks for work-up and intervention seems unwarranted. Some authors would also argue that because 66 percent of patients should have symptoms resolve within 2 weeks, work-up and possible intervention are warranted at the 2-week mark or earlier after discussion with the patient about symptoms, level of bother and willingness to risk possible intervention.

In our practice, if a patient is unable to void spontaneously (i.e. urinary retention) within 1 week after a retropubic or transobturator tape procedure, we consider and discuss loosening the sling at that time, provided that a simultaneous pelvic organ prolapse repair was not done. The work-up should include a focused history, physical examination, cystourethroscopy and urodynamic testing in selected cases. Key points in the history are the patient's preoperative voiding status and the temporal relationship of new symptoms to the surgical procedure for SUI. Physical examination should focus on the angulations of the urethra. The urethra should be evaluated to determine if it appears to be hypersuspended and whether the urethral meatus appears to be pulled toward the pubic bone because a more vertical angle of the urethra suggests obstruction. However, most patients after synthetic midurethral sling procedures do not appear overcorrected. Patients should be examined for prolapse, urethral hypermobility and recurrent SUI.

History

Preoperative voiding status and postoperatively development of new symptoms

As previously mentioned, cystourethroscopy should be performed to rule out any sling material in the urethra or bladder and to evaluate for any scarring, narrowing, occlusion, kinking, or deviation. It is also helpful to rule out any unsuspected pathology, such as a urethral diverticulum or bladder lesion.

Examination

- *Angulation of urethra*
- *Hypersuspended urethra*
- *Urethral meatus pulled towards pubic bone*

Urodynamics testing can be performed if there is doubt regarding the diagnosis based on history, physical examination and noninvasive testing (uroflow or post-void residual). There are no universally accepted urodynamics criteria for bladder outlet obstruction. Classic high pressure—low flow voiding dynamics confirm the diagnosis but are not always present even with significant obstruction owing to the differing voiding dynamics in women compared with men. For patients with complete retention shortly after surgery, urodynamics is of minimal diagnostic benefit. In a patient with retention, urodynamics can be used to identify detrusor instability, impaired compliance and confirm the diagnosis of obstruction. For a patient with predominately *de novo* storage symptoms with normal emptying, urodynamics can help identify or rule out obstruction. In these situations, many clinicians believe videourodynamics is preferable to standard urodynamics because the site of obstruction can be identified by fluoroscopy regardless of pressure and flow dynamics.

Urodynamics

- *Bladder outlet obstruction—high pressure low flow*
- *Postoperative retention—detrusor instability and obstruction*

Immediate Postoperative Retention after Retropubic Synthetic Midurethral Sling

Discussion

Cystourethroscopy

- *Mesh erosion*
- *Scarring*
- *Narrowing*
- *Occlusion*
- *Kinking*
- *Deviation*
- *Urethral*

Initially after incontinence surgery, there is a significant degree of swelling around the bladder and urethra. The swelling disrupts the nerve supply to the bladder which in turn makes it difficult to relax the urethra and initiate voiding. It may take anywhere from several days to several weeks for this swelling to clear. An inability to void after 2 or 3 weeks is most often due to external compression of the urethra. In other words, the tissue or material used to support the urethra is compressing the urethra at rest or with minimal straining. Sometimes the surgical tissues stretch over time and this compression relaxes.

In women with postoperative urinary retention after retropubic and transobturator synthetic midurethral sling procedures, we advocate early intervention (within 7 to 14 days after surgery) because most patients should be able to void spontaneously within 72 hours. Early sling loosening allows one to perform a minimally invasive procedure under local anesthesia in the office setting or operating room. The goal is to stretch or loosen the sling maintaining the suburethral continuity of the sling material. Most likely cutting the sling during an early intervention such as this would result in a higher probability of recurrent stress incontinence. When the sling is firmly adherent to the posterior urethra, great care must be taken not to injure the urethra when loosening the sling.

Technique for Synthetic Sling Loosening in the Acute Setting (7 to 14 Days)

- The patient is positioned in the lithotomy position and the vagina is prepared in a sterile fashion.
- The anterior vaginal wall is infiltrated with local anesthetic.

- The surgeon cuts the suture used to close the vaginal wall and opens the prior incision.
- The surgeon identifies the sling and hooks it with a right-angled clamp or other small clamp.
- The surgeon spreads the clamp or applies downward traction to loosen the tape 1 to 2 cm.
- The incision is closed with running absorbable suture. This technique is suitable to be performed in the office in a cooperative patient. However, it can be done in the operating room with very light intravenous sedation and local anesthesia in patients who are extremely anxious or intolerant of pain. It is best to perform this procedure before 14 days because after this time tissue in growth may prevent loosening, in which case it would most likely be preferable to cut the sling.

Takedown of Retropubic Synthetic Midurethral Sling at Four Months Postoperatively due to Voiding Dysfunction

Discussion

Up to 20 percent of women can have an extended period (up to 6 months) before being able to void without a self-catheterization or having to have an indwelling urinary catheter. The incidence of voiding dysfunctions goes up with age, being 12 percent under age 50 and as high as 50 percent over age 65. Six months is usually the cut-off that many doctors use because there can be a natural loosening that takes place up until then. After six months, it is unlikely that the obstructive symptoms will improve on their own, but in several series, the average time elapsed between the initial surgery and subsequent surgical takedown of the compressed urethra is as much as 14 to 18 months. Some physicians feel that if a woman is unable to void spontaneously by 8 weeks that there is urethral obstruction present and surgical revision should be considered. Other physicians will not consider surgical revision (urethrolysis) until at least 6 months have passed. Even if a woman can void on her own but with some difficulty, there can often be irritative bladder symptoms in which the detrusor muscle has spasms when it senses fullness. With high bladder volumes and bladder spasms, a woman may still need surgery to relieve urethral obstruction even though she can void without self catheterization.

In this case, a synthetic sling was placed too tightly and resulted in voiding dysfunction. When managing occult incontinence, we prefer to use a transobturator or a single-incision sling because the literature seems to indicate there is a slightly higher risk for voiding dysfunction after a retropubic synthetic sling. However, this remains an area of controversy because more recent literature has noted that occult incontinence is more common in patients with pelvic organ prolapse than had previously been thought. The keys to success of takedown of a synthetic sling revolve around successfully identifying the sling and mobilizing it completely away from the entire urethra. We have seen numerous situations in which the sling is simply cut in the midline and the voiding dysfunction persists.

Steps for Takedown of a Synthetic Midurethral Sling (Figures 16.1 and 16.2)

- Repeat cystourethroscopy is performed in the operating room to ensure there is no evidence of sling penetration in the urethra or bladder.
- Hydrodistention of the distal part of the anterior vaginal wall as previously described is performed.

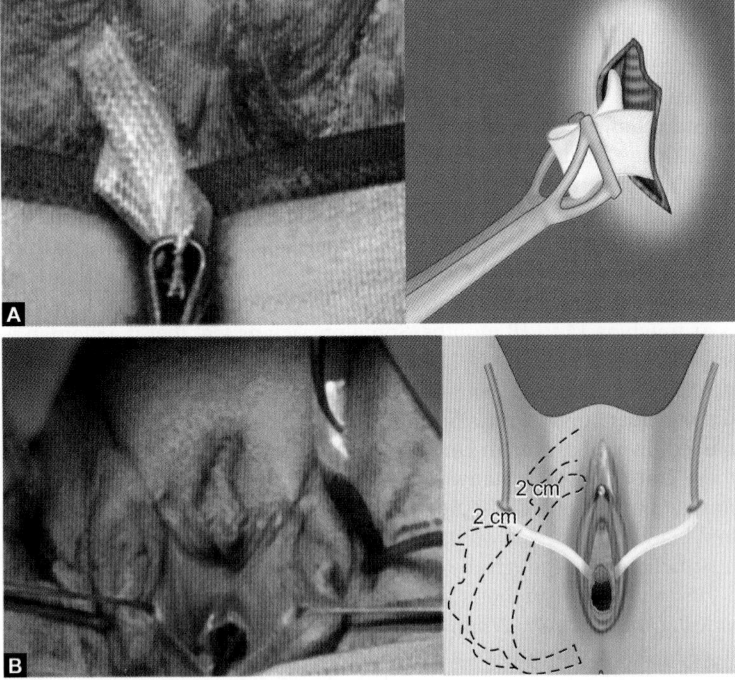

Figures 16.1A and B: Takedown of synethic midurethral sling

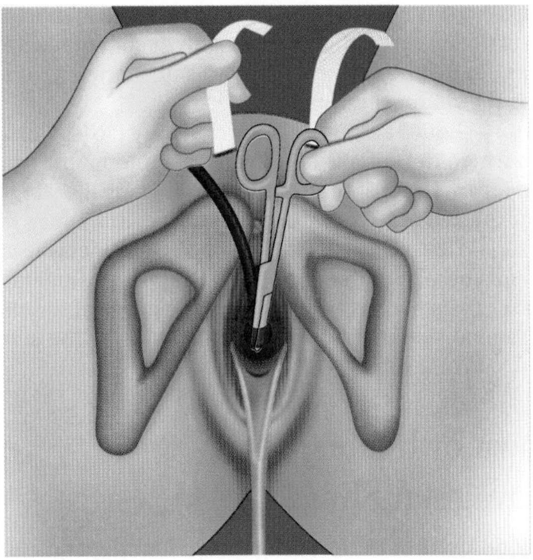

Figure 16.2: Tension-free placement of synethic midurethral sling

- A midline vertical anterior vaginal wall incision is made with a scalpel and the incision is taken down through the full thickness of the anterior vaginal wall. A gritty feeling detected with the knife indicates the location of the synthetic sling, appropriately identifying the location of the sling. If there is no gritty feeling detected with a knife, the tip of a finger can be used to palpate the area aggressively feeling for the synthetic polypropylene fibers. Frequently, the sling can be encased in scar tissue and can be under significant tension making it difficult to identify. A cystoscope or urethral sound can also be placed in the urethra with upward traction to help expose the exact location of the sling, isolating the axes of tension and indentation on the undersurface of the urethra.
- After the sling is identified, we prefer to cut it in the midline with scissors and sharply lyze it away from the urethra all the way back to the inferior pubic ramus on each side. Another technique involves passing a right-angled clamp between the urethra and the sling, placing a clamp on each side of the exposed sling and cutting it in the midline and then completing the lysis. If the sling is extremely tight, it can be isolated lateral to the urethra to avoid urethral injury. The mobilization of the sling off the urethra is only to the level of the endopelvic fascia; this preserves lateral support of the urethra because the retropubic space is not entered and it is hoped the likelihood of recurrent SUI is decreased.

- Surgeons should always obtain pathologic confirmation of the lysed portion of the synthetic sling because this documents a portion of the sling was cut in case the procedure was unsuccessful in completely resolving the voiding dysfunction.
- The urethra should always be inspected very closely for any injury. In cases where the sling is deep to the periurethral fascia, it can be ingrown into the wall of the urethra and excising the sling may result in an unexpected urethrotomy. In the event of this injury, the urethral defect should be closed in layers with a fine delayed-absorbable suture and the bladder continuously drained postoperatively for 7 to 10 days. The sling has been cut and the edges of the sling remain on the vaginal side of the urogenital diaphragm. The sling must be adjusted, cut, or taken down.

Takedown of Rectus Fascia in Pubovaginal Sling

The technique used to perform this procedure depends on the sling material and how it interacts with the patient's tissue. Certain autologous or allograft slings may aggressively incorporate with the surrounding tissue making it impossible to differentiate the sling material from the patient's tissue. In contrast, certain other biologic materials may be easily identifiable and easily dissected away from the patient's tissues and this is often unknown until the time of surgery. Whether or not the patient redevelops SUI or maintains continence is based on the degree of scarification, how aggressive the takedown is and what sling material is used. There is significant release of tension around the urethra when the sling is cut in the midline.

Retropubic and Vaginal Urethrolysis After Retropubic Suspension

A 75-year-old woman with a long-standing history of fairly severe urinary urgency, frequency and urge incontinence with recurrent urinary tract infection (UTI), atleast three documented urinary tract infections per year for the last several years. Antimuscarinic agents, have failed to improve her overactive bladder symptoms. She had undergone a previous retropubic urethral suspension approximately 10 years before presentation. On pelvic examination, the urethra is noted to be markedly elevated and fixed with no bladder neck mobility. Post-void residual measurements are consistently between 200 and

300 mL. Cystourethroscopy notes a normal urethra and bladder. Videourodynamics testing is performed and notes obvious detrusor overactivity with voluntary voiding pressures of 42 cm H_2O with a maximum flow rate of 8 mL/s. There is an obvious area of obstruction caused by over elevation at the level of the proximal urethra.

Based on the diagnosis of refractory detrusor overactivity in the face of outlet urethral obstruction and incomplete bladder emptying, urethrolysis is discussed and recommended. Both a vaginal and retropubic urethrolysis would be reasonable options. In this case, a better outcome most likely would occur from a retropubic takedown because the previous suspension is done retropubically. However, this is a controversial topic with the ultimate decision left to the discretion of the surgeon and his or her own clinical experience and expertise regarding urethrolysis.

In general, the surgery to release urethral obstruction is about 85 to 90 percent successful to the point that a woman does not need to self-catheterize or have an indwelling Foley's catheter, but there is a new or recurrence of stress incontinence rate of about 10 to 20 percent. Thus the total success of the procedure is about 65 to 80 percent.

Both Techniques for Urethrolysis Retropubic or Abdominal Vesicourethrolysis

- A large Foley's catheter with a 30 mL balloon is placed inside the bladder.
- A transverse incision (preferably Cherney's incision) is performed to facilitate exposure into the retropubic space.
- The bladder is taken down sharply off the back of the symphysis pubis all the way down the proximal urethra. It is best to make a high cystotomy to help in this dissection. It is important to mobilize the bladder and the proximal urethra completely from the back of the symphysis. The sutures or bone anchors from the previous suspension commonly are encountered and cut.
- Dissection is extended laterally toward the pelvic sidewall and is taken down the level of the origin of the arcus tendineus fasciae pelvis or white line. This is also the lower margin of the obturator internus fascia.
- When there is significant concern of rescarification of this area, it is sometimes beneficial to make a window in the peritoneum and bring a piece of omentum if available through the window to be placed between the back of the symphysis and the proximal urethra. Resuspension is almost never necessary. If a high cystocele is present in conjunction with the obstruction from the bladder neck suspension, a retropubic paravaginal defect repair can be performed simultaneously with the takedown.

Technique for Cherney Muscle-cutting Incision

- A finger is taken around the entire belly of the rectus muscle. The finger should be behind the rectus muscle and in front of the peritoneum. The insertion of the muscle is taken off the back of the symphysis via electrocautery.
- The muscle has been completely detached from its insertion.
- Easy access to the retropubic space is apparent after both rectus muscles have been cut.

Technique of Retropubic Vesicourethrolysis

- A high extraperitoneal cystotomy has been made to facilitate sharp dissection of the bladder of the back of the symphysis pubis.
- Sharp dissection is continued down in the midline until the proximal one-third of the urethra has been mobilized off the symphysis.
- Dissection is extended laterally down to the level of the paravaginal attachment at the arcus tendineus fasciae pelvis (White line).
- To prevent rescarification in this area, a piece of omentum can be brought through a window in the peritoneum. The omentum is sutured at the midline to the lower aspect of the symphysis and laterally to the obturator fascia with numerous delayed-absorbable sutures.

Technique for Vaginal Urethrolysis

- A transurethral Foley's catheter with a 30 mL balloon is placed within the bladder. Initial traction on the catheter with simultaneous vaginal palpation of bladder neck subjectively assesses the degree and extent of scarring elevation and fixation of the proximal urethra and bladder neck. The goal of vaginal urethrolysis is to create some mobility at the proximal urethra and bladder neck.
- An 'inverted-U' incision is made and the vaginal wall is dissected off the underlying urethra and bladder neck. Allis clamps are used to grab the lateral part of the vaginal incision and the dissections are extended laterally toward the inferior pubic ramus on each side.
- Perforation of the urogenital diaphragm is performed using curved Mayo scissors pointing toward the ipsilateral shoulder. The tips of the scissors should penetrate the urogenital diaphragm at the inferior border of the inferior pubic ramus. The scissors are separated and usually a finger is inserted and blunt takedown of all attachments of the urethra and bladder to the sidewall is performed bilaterally. Urethral mobility is subjectively assessed via traction on the Foley's catheter. The dissection is continued until some urethral mobility has been created.
- The entire area is irrigated, hemostasis is controlled and the vaginal incision is closed usually with interrupted delayed-absorbable sutures.

Postoperative Care after Sling Revision or Takedown

In most cases after sling loosening or incision, the patient is sent home without a catheter and is given perioperative antibiotics only. The patient should void before leaving the office or recovery room. A catheter is left *in situ* in the event of urethral injury during sling incision or loosening or in cases of extensive urethrolysis. The length of catheterization depends on the size and nature of the injury and can range from 3 to 14 days. For patients who are hospitalized after transvaginal or retropubic urethrolysis, a vaginal packing and Foley's catheter are left in overnight and the catheter is left in place until vaginal packing is removed or until discharge if the patient is unable to void spontaneously while in the hospital. Ideally, the patient is instructed to perform clean intermittent catheterization, but if she is unwilling or unable, a Foley's catheter is reinserted.

Outcomes

Very few objective data are available in the published literature regarding the results after sling loosening of synthetic midurethral slings. The few data available seem to indicate that such an intervention in these patients leads to resolution of their symptoms in 80 to 100 percent of cases. Resolution of voiding symptoms after sling incision has been reported to occur in 70 to 100 percent of cases, regardless of the type of sling. Resolution of voiding symptoms after transvaginal urethrolysis for all types of slings has been reported to be 33 to 92 percent. Time to intervention in all of these series was different and this may play a role in the ultimate success of the intervention. Patient bother, morbidity of procedure, type of anti-incontinence procedure and the patient's willingness to risk recurrent SUI should determine timing and treatment options. SUI after sling loosening, sling incision and transvaginal urethrolysis is a complication that should be discussed with all patients before intervention. The reported rates vary greatly and the true rates are likely unknown owing to underreporting. Incidence of SUI after sling loosening, sling incision, or urethrolysis ranges from 0 to 39 percent with varying degrees of follow-up. We generally counsel patients by telling them they have a 15 to 30 percent chance of recurrence of SUI based on timing and type of takedown or sling revision.

Conclusion

Voiding dysfunction and/or retention occurs in the best of hands in a small percentage of patients after procedures to correct SUI.

Ultimate timing and type of intervention for these problems should be individualized in the hope of meeting the patient's needs.

Bibliography

1. Alcalay M, Monga A, Stanton SL. Burch colposuspension: a 10-20 year follow-up. Br J Obstet Gynaecol. 1995;102(9):740-5.
2. Barber MD, Kleeman S, Karram MM, et al. Transobturator tape compared with tension-free vaginal tape for the treatment of stress urinary incontinence. Obstet Gynecol. 2008;111(3):611-21.
3. Campeau L, Al-Afraa T, Corcos J. Evaluation and management of urinary retention after a suburethral sling procedure in women. Curr Urol Rep. 2008;9(5):412-8.
4. Cross CA, Cespedes RD, English SF, et al. Transvaginal urethrolysis for urethral obstruction after anti-incontinence surgery. J Urol. 1998;159(4):1199-201.
5. Filbeck T, Ullrich T, Pichlmeier U, Kiel HJ, Wieland WF, Roessler W. Correlation of persistent stress urinary incontinence with quality of life after suspension procedures: is continence the only decisive postoperative criterion of success? Urology. 1999;54(2):247-51.
6. Guerette NL, Bena JF, Davila GW. Transobturator slings for stress incontinence: using urodynamic parameters to predict outcomes. Int Urogynecol J. 2008;19(1):97-102.
7. Karram MM, Segal JL, Vassallo BJ, et al. Complications and untoward effects of the tension-free vaginal tape procedure. Obstet Gynecol. 2003;101(5 Pt 1):929-32.
8. Klutke C, Siegel S, Carlin B, et al. Klutke Urinary retention after tension-free vaginal tape procedure: incidence and treatment. J Urol. 2001;58(5):697-701.
9. Maher CF, Dwyer PL, Carey MP, et al. Colposuspension or sling for low urethral pressure stress incontinence? Int Urogynecol J Pelvic Floor Dysfunct. 1999;10(6):384-9.
10. Morgan TO Jr, Westney OL, McGuire EJ. Pubovaginal sling: 4-year outcome analysis and quality of life assessment. J Urol. 2000;163(6):1845-8.
11. Nager CW, Siris L, Litman HJ, et al. Baseline urodynamic predictors of treatment failure 1 year after midurethral sling surgery. J Urol. 2011;186:597-603.
12. Parys BT, Haylen BT, Hutton JL, et al. The effects of simple hysterectomy on vesicourethral function. Br J Urol. 1989;64(6):594-9.
13. Walters MD, Karram MM. Urogynecology and Reconstructive Pelvic Surgery, 3rd edn. Philadeplhia: Mosby, 2007.
14. Wein AJ, Kavoussi LR, Novick AC, et al, (Eds). Campbell-Walsh Urology, 10th edn. Philadelphia, PA: Elsevier Saunders; 2011:chap 73.

CHAPTER

17

Complications, Difficulties and Redo Procedure for Stress Urinary Incontinence Surgeries

Madhuri Gandhi, Sarika Dodwani, Prakash Trivedi

Introduction

There are no surgeries without complications, difficulties and failures. Urinary incontinence surgeries are no exception. We will describe issues with all surgical procedures.

Laparoscopic Burch

Serious complications are rare with this type of surgery. However, no surgery is without risk and the main potential complications are listed below:

- Intraoperative blood loss requiring transfusion <1 percent.
- Damage to the bowel, bladder or bladder requiring further surgery <1 percent. The bowel can be easily prevented from intraoperative injury with proper preoperative bowel preparation. If there is any doubt of bladder or urethral injury, it can be confirmed by cystoscopy in the same sitting.
- Urinary tract infections and wound infections can occur in 5 percent of patients which can be prevented by proper antibiotic cover in perioperative period.
- Failure rate of 10 to 15 percent. In a patient with recurrent or persistent incontinence after previous operation, the patient should undergo a complete evaluation which should also include cystourethroscopy. Because sometimes in a case of urethral diverticulum, the patient can leak secondary to overflow of urine from the urethral diverticulum during stress provocation. In this case a repeat sling procedure will not be beneficial.
- There are chances of developing urgency, or urge incontinence after the operation in 5 percent of the cases. Proper case selection can avoid such complications.

- Difficulty emptying the bladder that necessitates prolonged self-catheterization in 1 percent of the subjects
- Thrombotic episodes though rare can occur in <1 percent patients. It is worth considering thromboprophylactic measures for the patients with various risk factors for thrombotic episodes
- The development of new vaginal prolapse, i.e. enterocele after the operation in 10 to 16 percent. We recommend to do McCall's culdoplasty also with colposuspension to avoid postoperative enterocele.
- Less than one percent may experience long-term pubic pain
- Conversion from the laparoscopic to the open surgery is done in <1 percent cases, reasons being poor case selection and less expertise.

Though open Burch surgery is done by many and it is still having the place, laparoscopic Burch has few difficulties like need of instrumentation and need of skills, difficult laparoscopic suturing.

Tension-free Vaginal Tape, Trivedi's Stress Urinary Incontinence Tape (TSUIT) and Suburethral Sling

Though the tension-free vaginal tape (TVT) sling is considered a standard sling surgery today, complications can still occur. It is very important to note that it typically is not the mesh itself or the procedure that is the cause of the complication, it is how the mesh is placed or how the body heals around the mesh that is the underlying cause.

Difficulties

- Avoiding bladder while passing TVT needle and use metal guard while passing catheter. Bladder perforation at the time of retropubic synthetic sling placement occurs in almost 3 to 5 percent of cases **(Figure 17.1)**. The needle almost always perforates the bladder high up between 1 and 3 o'clock position on the left side and 9 o'clock and 11 o'clock position on the right side. Because the site of penetration is usually high up in the nondependent portion of the bladder and the diameter of the needle is quite small (3–5 mm), it has been our experience that continuous postoperative drainage is not required. However in certain situation we would recommend drainage for few days to a week (i.e. if multiple perforations occur, if there is significant hematuria or if the perforation was low in the base of bladder).
- Retropubic space bleeding can occur as numerous vessels can be injured during the blind passage of retropubic midurethral sling (MUS) trocar including the vessels in the wall of vagina (veins of Santorini), abberant obturator vessels, and obturator neurovascular bundle **(Figure 17.2)**. The retopubic space is generally a very forgiving

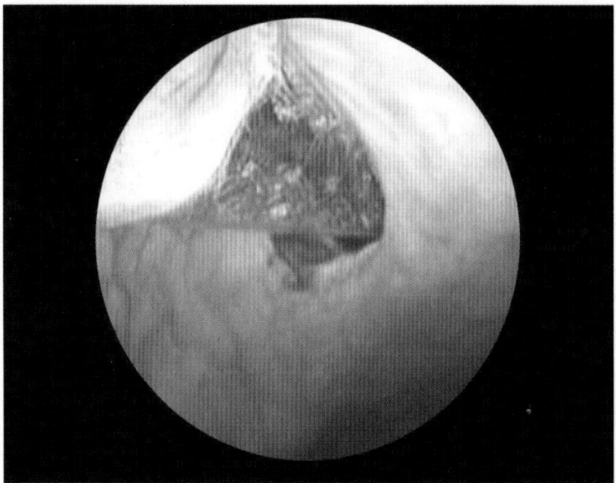

Figure 17.1: Bladder perforation during TVT/T-SUIT

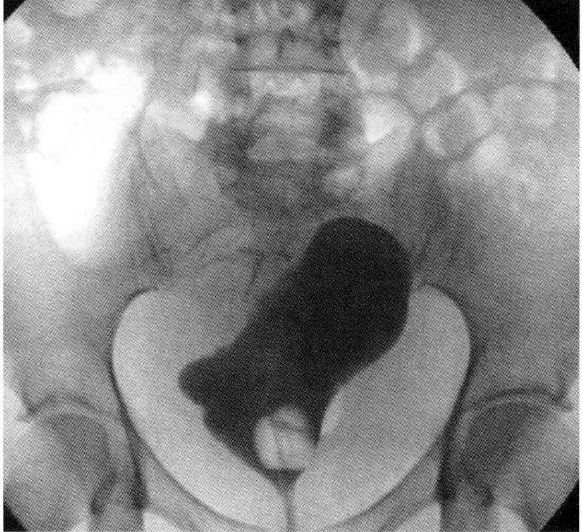

Figure 17.2: Cystogram showing massive retropubic hematoma

space and stable hematomas usually resolve without complications, however in patients whose condition do not stabilize, exploratory laparotomy would be required considering a major vessel injury.

- Higher chance of retention

Complications

- Mesh erosion into the bladder **(Figure 17.3)** and in vagina **(Figure 17.4)**.

If this occurs, this can cause bladder pain, recurrent bladder or urinary tract infections (UTIs), blood in the urine, or other urinary symptoms

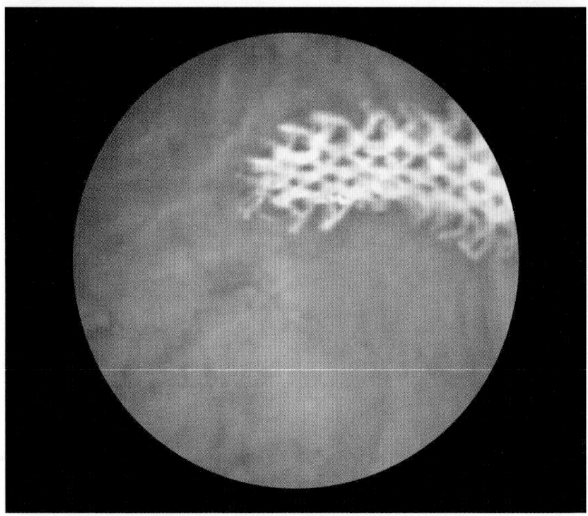

Figure 17.3: Mesh erosion in bladder

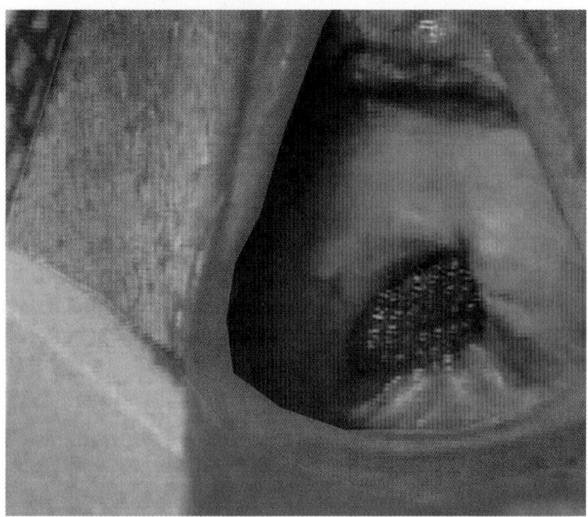

Figure 17.4: Mesh erosion in vagina

such as frequency, urgency, or painful urination. If a patient is having these symptoms, cystoscopy should be completed to ensure that the mesh has not eroded into the bladder. If the mesh is in the bladder, it will need to be removed. The mesh can be removed laparoscopically.

A finding of persistent granulation tissue and bleeding from vagina, indicates the presence of ongoing reaction between the foreign body and the surrounding tissue, and complete excision of the tape is usually required. This occurs when nontype 1 macroporus mesh is used.

- *Calcification of eroded mesh (Figures 17.5A and B):* This is a rare complication. The mesh needs to be removed.
- *Mesh infection or abscess formation:* This is a very rare complication. Typically the entire mesh tape needs to be removed.
- Tension-free vaginal tape track fistula containing mesh sometimes causes pain and has to be removed by excision **(Figures 17.6A and B)**
- *Urinary obstructive symptoms:* If any sling is placed too tight, it can cause urinary retention or various amounts of incomplete emptying syndromes. The patient may complain of dribbling micturition or an intermittent dribbling or complete urinary retention. Most will agree that the postvoid residual (the amount of urine in the bladder after voiding) should be less than 100 or 125 cc (about 3 oz). If the amount in the bladder is higher than this, then the sling could be too tight. It can also cause symptoms such as urgency, frequency and feeling the bladder is just not emptying. If this is found to be the cased, the sling needs to be loosened or released.
- *Vaginal and/or abdominal pain:* Occasionally, the mesh will heal in a way, or was placed in a way that causes vaginal and/or abdominal pain and can occur in less than 1 percent of cases. If the mesh is irritating a nerve in the abdominal wall, or is too tight or pulling

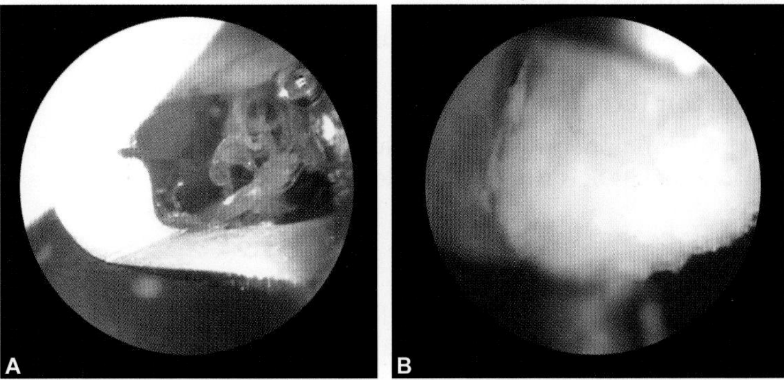

Figures 17.5A and B: Calcification of eroded mesh

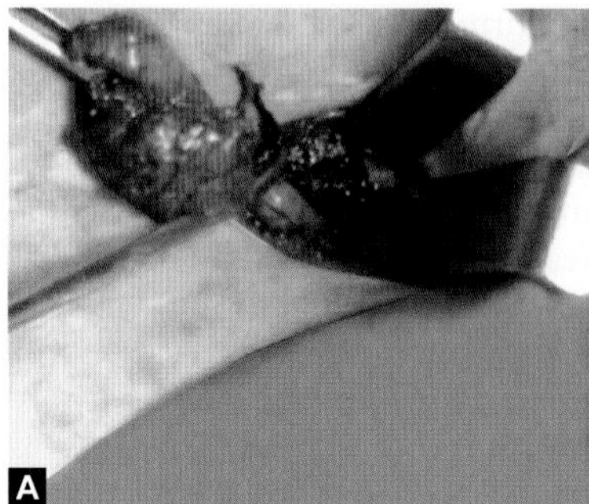

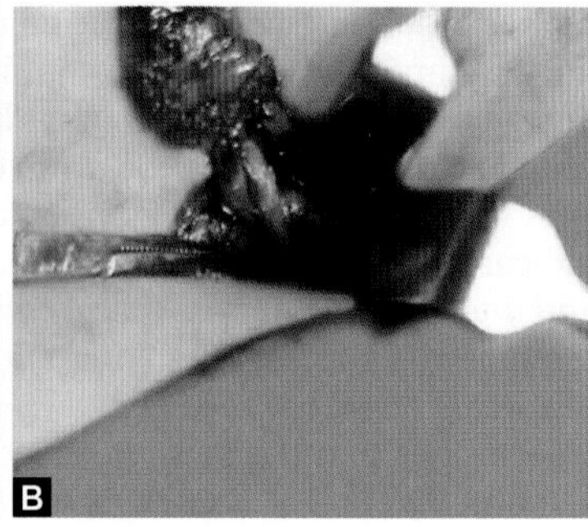

Figures 17.6A and B: TVT track fistula with mesh and its excision

on the abdominal wall or vagina, this can cause significant pain during normal daily activities or with intercourse. If the pain is just vaginally with intercourse, this can sometimes be approached with just a vaginal procedure and removing or releasing the mesh through a small vaginal incision. However, if the pain is in the abdomen or bladder as well, most of the time the entire sling will need to be removed by a laparoscopic approach.

Tension-free Vaginal Tape-Obturator, Trivedi Obturator Tape and Trivedi Obturator Tape Adjustable

Outside in Techniques

General lesser complications, difficulties but few failures.

Inside Out Techniques

1. More chronic pain in thighs and legs.
2. Occasionally, it can have some bleeding.

Mini Arc

Though the procedure is simple but long-term results are not known. May have less morbidity but there can be failures.

Bulking Agents

Injectable therapy using bulking agents composed of synthetic materials, bovine collagen, or an autologous substance augments the urethral wall and increases urethral resistance to urinary flow. Injection of bulking agents to treat a dysfunctional urethra is a minimally invasive method of correcting intrinsic sphincteric deficiency (ISD) that results in stress urinary incontinence (SUI).

Complications are rare. Polytetrafluoroethylene (PTFE) paste is not used because of migration from local site. There might be reaction with the bulking agent.

- Bulking agents give temporary relief.
- Bulking agents are costly.

Artificial Urethral Sphincter

Intraoperative Complications

The balloon reservoir is placed intra-abdominally or in an extraperitoneal prevesical space (space of Retzius). Iatrogenic peritoneotomy and bowel injury have been reported. Injury to the urethra, vagina, and rectum. Vaginal injuries are closed primarily. If a rectal injury occurs, the procedure must be abandoned.

Postoperative complications can be described as mechanical or nonmechanical. The reported reoperation rate for the artificial urinary sphincter is 17 to 35 percent, with about 50 percent of these cases caused by mechanical complications and 50 percent by nonmechanical complications.

- *Mechanical complications:* Mechanical failure caused by loss of fluid from the system. It can also occur because of obstruction of flow due to debris, airlock, blood, or crystallized material.
- *Nonmechanical complications:*
  - *Infection:* The overall risk of infection is reported to be 2 to 3 percent for initial artificial urinary
  - *Tissue atrophy:* A common cause of recurrent stress incontinence is loss of cuff compression due to tissue atrophy. Tissue atrophy is the most common cause of nonmechanical failure and has been reported to be the most common cause of surgical revision. Tissue atrophy results from local tissue ischemia around the cuff.
  - *Overactive bladder (OAB) syndrome: De novo* symptoms of OAB, such as urgency, frequency, nocturia, and urgency incontinence, may develop in up to 23 percent of patients who did not have these symptoms preoperatively.

- *Cuff erosion:* One of the most feared complications of the artificial urinary sphincter is cuff erosion. Cuff erosion most commonly occurs within 3 to 4 months after surgery. The artificial urethral sphincters are costly.

Bibliography

1. Azam U, Frazer MI, Kozman EL, et al. The tension-free vaginal tape procedure in women with previous failed stress incontinence surgery. J Urol. 2001;166:554-6.
2. Fa lagas ME, Velakoulis S, Iavazzo C, Athanasiou S. Mesh-related infections after pelvic organ prolapse repair surgery. Eur J Obstet Gynecol Reprod Biol. 2007;134:147-56.
3. Kolle D, Tamussino K, Hanzal E, et al. Bleeding complications with the tension-free vaginal tape operation. Am J Obstet Gynecol. 2005;193: 2045-49.
4. Latthe PM, Singh P, Foon R, Toozs-Hobson P. Two routes of transobturator tape procedures in stress urinary incontinence: a meta-analysis with direct and indirect comparison of randomized trials. BJU Int. 2010;106:68-76.
5. Long CY, Hsu CS, Wu MP, Liu CM, Wang TN, Tsai EM. Comparison of tension-free vaginal tape and transobturator tape procedure for the treatment of stress urinary incontinence. Curr Opin Obstet Gynecol. 2009;21:342-7.
6. Rehder P, Glodny B, Pichler R, Mitterberger MJ. Massive retropubic hematoma after minimal invasive mid-urethral sling procedure in a patient with a corona mortis. Indian J Urol (2010).
7. Sokol AI, Jelousek JE, Walters MD, et al. Incidence and predictors of prolonged urinary retention after TVT with and without concurrent prolapse surgery. Am J Obstet Gynecol. 2005;192:1537-43
8. Tsivian A, Kessler O, Mogutin B, et al. Tape related complications of the tension-free vaginal tape procedure. J Urol. 2004;171:2762-4.
9. Wang KH, Neimark M, Davila GW. Voiding dysfunction following TVT procedure. Int Urogynecol J Pelvic Floor Dysfunct. 2002;13:353-7, discussion 358.

CHAPTER

18

Bulking Agents

S Mahadevan

Background

Injectable bulking agents have been used to treat female stress urinary incontinence (FSUI) and correcting intrinsic sphincter deficiency (ISD) over the last 15 years.

These agents augment the urethral wall and increase the urethral resting tone to urinary flow.[1-3]

The agents used are autologous fat, bovine collagen, calcium hydroxylapatite, carbon bead particles, dextranomer/hyaluronic copolymer (Zuidex) polytetrafluoroethylene paste, and polydimethylsiloxane **(Table 18.1)**.

Ongoing development, research and trials continue to provide evidence based experience with this form of minimally invasive treatment of FSUI.

National Institute for Health and Clinical Excellence (NICE) has issued guidelines on the use of bulking agents in 2005.[4]

Indications

- In patients where surgical treatment by tension-free vasinal tape (TVT)/transobturator tape (TOT) are contraindicated because of severe morbidity
- Patients choice
- Contraindications to anesthesia
- In failed cases of surgery for stress incontinence where there is severe scarring of urethral and paraurethral tissues
- In intrinsic sphincter deficiency (ISD).

Table 18.1: Bulking agents

Agent	*Properties*	*Mode of action*	*Type of anesthesia*	*Adverse effects*	*Efficacy*
Autologous fat[5]	Ideal, inexpensive, non-allergenic—harvested from patient's abdominal wall	Local acting bulks the urethra	GA as fat has to be harvested from abdominal wall	Abdominal pain and infection at site of liposuction	Good results short term only as eventually phagocytosis of fat
Bovine collagen (Contigen)[6]	Bovine collagen purified and cross linked with glutaraldehyde	Injected collagen is replaced by host collagen over a year	Can be performed in outpatient setting under LA	Allergic reaction Skin testing 4 to 6 weeks prior to procedure	Lasts 6 to 12 months
Calcium hydroxyapatite(CH) (Coaptite)[7]	Particles of CH with sodium carboxy-methyl cellulose	Promote tissue growth and new collagen formation	Outpatient under LA	No prior skin testing	Efficacy greater than bovine collagen Effects wear off after 1 year
Carbon bead particles (Durasphere)[8]	Nonbiodegradable particles	Locally acting to promote fibrosis and support	Can be injected under LA increased viscosity needing wider gauge needle	Few	Effective 1 to 2 years
Dextranomer/ hyaluronic copolymer (Zuidex)[9]	Local bulking effect	Local action	LA via an injecter system implacer	Few	Not many studies available

Contd...

Contd...

Agent	***Properties***	***Mode of action***	***Type of anesthesia***	***Adverse effects***	***Efficacy***
Polytetrafluoroethylene paste (PTFE)[10]	Inert plastic material	Initiates foreign body reaction and granuloma formation	LA	Large bore needle required. Possibility of local and distant migration of particles into the lymph nodes, lung and brain	Good studies stopped because of side effects
Polydimethyl-siloxane (Macroplastique)[11]	Permanent material	Local bulking agent	LA	None	No long-term studies available Good results at 12 months

Contraindications

- Over active bladder (OAB)
- Limitation of a particular bulking agent because of allergy.

Preparation and Technique

Anesthesia: All agents can be injected under LA with or without additional sedation in the outpatient setting. Exception is the autologous fat injection where a general anesthesia is required. Fat is harvested from the patient's abdominal wall.

Technique

There are two methods to administer the bulking agent:
- *Transurethral technique:* Under cystoscopic guidance bladder neck is identified and the agent is injected into the submucosa of the urethra at this site under vision, till closure of the bladder neck is obtained. Confirmation of adequate bulking and closure of bladder neck can be achieved by cough test at this point.
- *Perurethral route:* Cystoscopy is done to identify the bladder neck. The needle is passed through the vagina and the bulking agent is injected into the submucosa at the level of bladder neck. Adequate bulking is ensured to close the bladder neck. A 0° cystoscope is usually used initially and subsequently a 30° and 70° scopes can be used to check correct all round placement.

Postoperative Care

All patients should be warned of possible urinary retention. They should be taught intermittent self catheterization (ISC) routinely. There is no need to insert Foleys catheter routinely.
Simple analgesia is all that is needed in majority of patients.

Complications—rare: Polytetrafluoroethylene (PTFE) is not used because of migration from local site as described above.

Efficacy: Almost all bulking agents are effective in the short-term. Re-injection may be required after 6 to 12 months (depending on the agent used)

Conclusion

Bulking agents are useful in the management of FSUI and ISD. They can be used in the outpatient setting except autologous fat injection. They have very few side effects and are easy to administer. They can be repeated. However, there is no single agent which has long-term effect. They are very useful adjuvant in the management of patients with stress in continence where surgical treatment is contraindicated.

Further research and clinical trials are ongoing with newer agents.

References

1. Benshushan A, Brzezinski A, Shoshani O. Periurethral injection for the treatment of urinary incontinence. Obstet Gynecol Surv. 1998; 53(6):383-8. [Medline].
2. Duckett JR. The use of periurethral injectables in the treatment of genuine stress incontinence. Br J Obstet Gynaecol. 1998;105(4):390-6. [Medline].
3. Keegan PE, Atiemo K, Cody J, et al. Periurethral injection therapy for urinary incontinence in women. Cochrane Database Syst Rev. 2007;(3):CD003881. [Medline].
4. National Institute for Health and Clinical Excellence-Intramural urethral bulking procedure for stress urinary incontinence in women: issue date Nov 2005, Interventional Procedure Guidance 138.
5. Su TH, Wang KG, Hsu CY. Periurethral fat injection in the treatment of recurrent genuine stress incontinence. J Urol. 1998;159(2):411-4. [Medline].
6. Gorton E, Stanton S, Monga A. Periurethral collagen injection: a long-term follow-up study. BJU Int. 1999; 84(9):966-71. [Medline].
7. Mayer RD, Dmochowski RR, Appell RA, et al. Multicenter prospective randomized 52-week trial of calcium hydroxylapatite versus bovine dermal collagen for treatment of stress urinary incontinence. Urology. 2007;69(5):876-80. [Medline].
8. Lightner D, Calvosa C, Andersen R. A new injectable bulking agent for treatment of stress urinary incontinence: results of a multicenter, randomized, controlled double-blind study of Durasphere. Urology. 2001;58(1):12-5. [Medline].
9. Chapple CR, Haab F, Cervigni M, et al. An open, multicentre study of NASHA/Dx Gel (Zuidex) for the treatment of stress urinary incontinence. Eur Urol. 2005; 48(3):488-94. [Medline].
10. Hidar S, Attyaoui F, de Leval J. Periurethral injection of silicone microparticles in the treatment of sphincter deficiency urinary incontinence. Prog Urol. 2000;10(2):219-23. [Medline].
11. Ghoniem G, Corcos J, Comiter C, et al. Cross-linked polydimethylsiloxane injection for female stress urinary incontinence: results of a multicenter, randomized, controlled single-blind study. J Urol. 2009;181(1):204-10. [Medline].

CHAPTER

19

Botulinum Toxin Injection Therapy

Animesh Gandhi, Yugali Warade, Prakash Trivedi

Introduction

Botulinum toxin is the most potent toxin known in the world. Through its neuromodulatory and paralytic mechanism, it has been applied to facial cosmesis, muscle and neurologic spasticity and migraine headaches. Its use for the treatment of voiding dysfunction has increased over the past several years and has had profound effects on patients with neurogenic bladder dysfunction and idiopathic detrusor overactivity (i.e. overactive bladder) when medical therapies fail. It is easy to use and is generally well-tolerated by the patient with the benefits usually outweighing the adverse events. At the present time botulinum toxin (BoTN) is approved by US Food and Drug Administration (US-FDA) for use in the genitor-urinary system for neurogenic bladder and FDA approval for idiopathic detrusor overactivity is expected in the near future.

Mechanism of Action

Depending on the serotype of the organism, *Clostridium botulinum,* seven distinct botulinum toxins can be produced by the bacterium (Types A, B, C1, D, E, F and G), all with similar mechanism of action. At the present time, only BoTN A **(Figure 19.1)** [Botox (Allergan, Irvine, CA) or Dysport (Medicis, Scottsdale, AZ)] and BoTN B [Myobloc or Neurobloc (Solstice Neuroscience, Louisvile, KY)] are commercially available for clinical use. BoTN acts by cleaving a specific site (specific to each BoTN serotype) of a protein complex [soluble N-ethylmaleimide-sensitive fusion protein attachment protein receptor (SNARE) complex] responsible for exocytosis of neurotransmitter vesicles from the neuron. In the case of BoTN A, the most well-studied toxin subtype, the specific substrate is the synaptosomal associated protein of 25 KD (SNAP-25), a component of SNARE complex, which results in the inhibition of

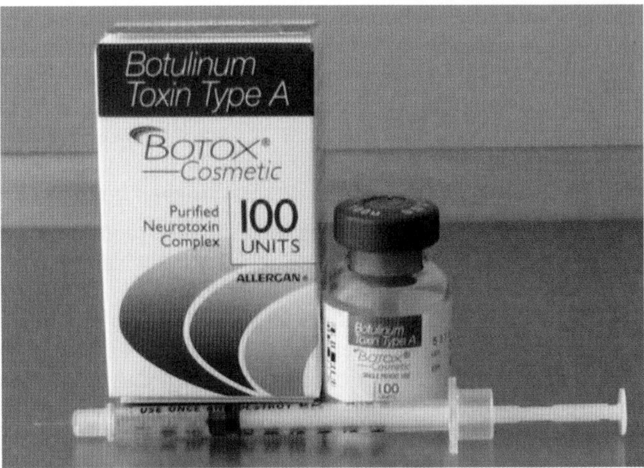

Figure 19.1: Botulinum A Toxin 100 units in powder form

synaptic release of acetylcholine from the peripheral motor neuron end plate at the neuromuscular junction and ensuing muscle paralysis. More recent experience also suggests toxin effect on neurotransmitters related to sensory function in the lower urinary tract.

- In normal neurotransmitter release at the neuromuscular junction, the synaptic fusion complex comprising the SNARE proteins mediates synaptic vesicle fusion to the acetylcholine exocytosis.
- In the presence of BoTN, which cleaves various SNARE proteins at sites specific to BoTN serotypes, the SNARE complex cannot form, and vesicle fusion and exocytosis is inhibited. At therapeutic doses of 100 to 300 units, BoTN A induces paralysis in the detrusor muscle. However, BoTN A may additionally inhibit sensory nerve activity directly and modulate bladder sensory transmission to the central nervous system. In the cases of bladder overactivity (both neurogenic and idiopathic) and in bladder compliance abnormalities, both mechanisms of action are exploited.

BoTN A specifically is a noncompetitive agonist, and as such the effects are irreversible yet also temporary as well. After administration of BoTN A, neuromuscular function regained primarily through a process of motor neuron end plate regeneration and sprouting of the distal motor nerve. The duration of the effect is variable, but in the bladder, the clinical response to BoTN A injections lasts approximately 6 months. The most common adverse event is increased postvoid residual volume, which can occur in 10 to 20 percent of patients undergoing injection. Cauterization may be required, and secondary urinary tract infection may ensue. More recent changes in BoTN A labeling, in response to systemic effects associated with toxin use in skeletal muscle, include warnings regarding systemic absorption of toxin and respiratory effects resulting from disseminated toxin effects.

Case Scenario

Very old woman has had severe urge incontinence requiring multiple pads per day for more than 3 years. She is neurologically intact with no other significant morbidities. Physical examination is normal, and urinalysis and cytology are negative. She received two different antimuscarinic agents, each for one month, with dose escalation being used. She had no significant reduction in symptoms despite medication combination and optimizing behavioral therapy. Urodynamics reveals a maximum bladder capacity of 175 mL, with detrusor overactivity occurring at 100 mL with incontinence. There is no evidence of obstructed voiding, and minimal postvoid residual is noted. Diagnostic cystoscopy is unremarkable. It is thought that this patient would be a good candidate for either neuromodulation or BoTN A injections. After risks and benefits of each of these therapies are discussed in great detail, the patient elects to proceed with BoTN A injections.

Botulinum Toxin Bladder Injection Technique

There is no standardized technique or approach to bladder injections of BoTN; a wide range of doses have been used, and many different injection templates have been followed. Generally, BoTN can be injected in the detrusor under direct cystoscopic guidance, with local or general anesthesia. A standard rigid or flexible cystourethroscope is used with a 23 gauge injection needle for toxin delivery. The effects of BoTN injection are apparent with symptom improvements noted within the first 7 to 10 days after injection. The therapeutic effects usually resolve after approximately 6 months, although after sequential injections (third or more) the beneficial effects may last longer (up to 9 months).

Because most clinical experience involves the use of BoTN A serotype, this discussion focuses on this toxin subtype. Dosing of BoTN is defined by units of biologic activity and neither interchangeable nor directly comparable with other BoTN types. BoTN A is supplied in 100 unit and 200 unit vials as a dessicated powder, which is reconstituted immediately before injection with injectable grade, preservative free normal saline. Dosing protocols vary and 50 to 300 units may be injected at a single session. Depending on the desired concentration of injection solution, 10 mL of injectable saline is used to dissolve each vial of BoTN A, and the solution is drawn up in appropriately sized syringes. Typically, injection of BoTN proceeds with 10 to 30 submucosal injection sites spread across the base and posterior wall of bladder, including or not including the trigone, and injection of 0.1 to 1 mL each of BoTN solution, depending on the concentration (approx 10 units per injection).

- *Patient position:* The patient is positioned in a standard dorsal lithotomy position and prepared sterilely in a fashion usual for cystoscopy. Per procedural antibiotics are administered.
- *Analgesia:* Local anesthetic is used, with 2 percent lignocaine jelly injected intraurethrally followed by intravesical instillation of 100 mL of 2 percent lignocaine solution. Dwell time for the solution should be at least 20 minutes.
- *BoTN solution reconstitution:* The desiccated powder is reconstituted with preservative-free, injectable grade 0.9 percent saline, as discussed previously.
- *Cystoscopy:* Cystourethroscopy is performed initially. In addition to noting any abnormality within the bladder, understanding the size and configuration of the bladder helps in planning the spacing of BoTN injections so as to cover as much of the bladder as possible. Ideally, approximately 10 to 30 injections should be used to deliver the BoTN, and the required volume should be taken into consideration during reconstitution. The trigone is not injected.
- *BoTN injection:* With the cystoscope in the bladder, the 23 gauge needle (with BoTN containing syringe attached) is advanced out of the tip of the scope and directed towards the desired injection location. Care should be taken to avoid inserting the needle through a visible blood vessel in the bladder mucosa because this can lead to bothersome bleeding. The needle is advanced into the submucosa approximately 0.5 cm; typically, there is a slight loss of resistance on entering the mucosa. Once positioned, the BoTN solution is gently injected, approximately 0.5 to 1 mL, depending on concentration. Injecting at appropriate depth is important to avoid extravasating BoTN through the bladder wall or depositing the BoTN too superficially within the bladder mucosa. Ideally, injecting the solution raises the overlying mucosa only minimally, avoiding large blebs on the mucosal surface. After delivery, the needle is withdrawn and repositioned at the next location, and the process is repeated **(Figure 19.2)**.
- The bladder is drained at the completion of toxin delivery and post-procedural instructions are given.

Outcomes and Complications

Of patients treated for overactive bladder symptoms with BoTN A bladder injections, 60 to 80 percent showed improvements in

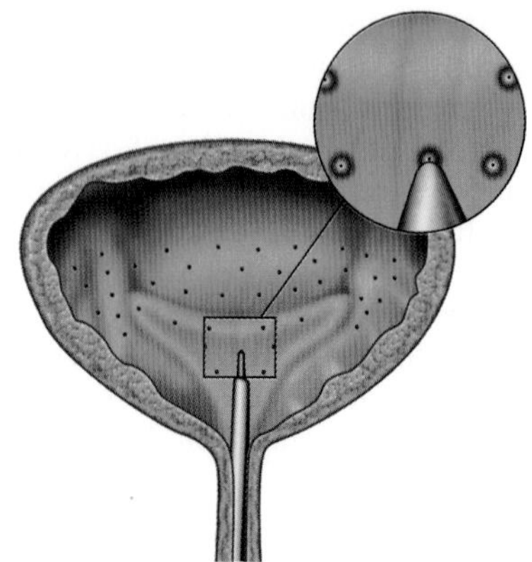

Figure 19.2: Multiple Botox A injections in bladder posterior wall

symptoms. Approximately, 70 percent of patient's neurogenic detrusor abnormalities have improvement. Efficacy is generally limited to 6 months because the effects abate as noted previously. Repeat injections can be performed with similar efficacy anticipated.

Controversy exists regarding whether or not the bladder trigone should be included in the injection template because there has been some theoretical concern of inducing vesicoureteral reflux by injecting near the uretheral orifices this concern has not been substantiated clinically. Because the trigone is thought to be densely innervated, many clinicians regularly include it in the template.

The major adverse event related to BoTN bladder injection is increased postvoid residual volume, which has been reported to occur approximately 10 to 20 percent of the time. Patients should be counseled regarding intermittent self-catheterization in the event that retention ensues. Retention is typically transient and resolves with time (usually ≤ 1 month). Minor complications of the procedure include transient dysuria, hematuria, and occasional urinary tract infection. More worrisome are rare reports of generalized weakness, and muscle weakness, possibly secondary to systemic effects of BoTN absorption.

Generally, the effect of BoTN A injection diminishes with time and abates by approximately 6 months after treatment. At this time, symptoms generally redevelop, and repeated injection is necessary to recoup any clinical benefit previously seen. With appropriate counseling, patients often are aware of this development and seek evaluation when they perceive the benefits are wearing off.

Botulinum toxin effect may be minimized in the presence of acute urinary tract infection, and urinary tract infection should be excluded before injection. Concomitant aminoglycoside administration at the time of toxin injection may obviate BoTN effect and should be avoided.

Injection depth should be optimized (entire needle point placed into the detrusor) to optimize therapy. Some patients may experience variability in response over sequential injections (the magnitude of efficacy effect may vary between injections), and individual undergoing repeat injections should be made aware of this possibility.

Increased urinary residual volume and urinary retention are the most common complications. This outcome can be mitigated by initial dosing at low levels and gradual increase of toxin dose overtime balancing effect and side effect to determine optimal individual dose magnitude.

Conclusion

With the FDA approval of BoTN for neurogenic causes of detrusor over activity and likely approval for idiopathic detrusor overactivity in the near future, the authors believe this therapy will be a good addition to the armamentarium of therapies available for this very common, very distressing problem.

Bibliography

1. Abdel-Meguid TA. Botulinum toxin—An injection into neurogenic overactive bladder—to include or exclude the trigone? A prospective, randomized controlled trial. J Urol. 2010;184(6):2423-8.
2. Anthony G, Brubaker, Linda, Richter, Holly E, et al. Anticholinergic Therapy vs on a botulinum toxin A for Urgency Urinary Incontinence New England Journal of Medicine. 2012;367(19):1803-13.
3. Digesu GA, Panayi D, Hendricken C, et al. Women's perspective of botulinum toxin treatment for overactive bladder symptoms. International Urogynecology Journal. 2011;22:425-31.
4. El-Khawand D, Wehbe S, Whitmore K. Botulinum toxin for conditions of the female pelvis. International Urogynecology Journal (Jan 2013);1433-3023 (MEDLINE from PubMed).
5. Jabs C, Carleton E. Efficacy of botulinum toxin A intradetrusor injections for non-neurogenic urinary urge incontinence: a randomized double-blind controlled trial. J Obstet Gynaecol Can. 2013;35(1):53-60.
6. Khan MS, Dasgupta P. Improvement in quality of life after botulinum toxin: an injection for idiopathic detrusor overactivity—results from a randomized double-blind placebo-controlled trial. BJU International. 2009.p.103.

CHAPTER

20

Sacral Nerve Stimulation

Ian P Tucker

Definition

- Neuromodulation is a treatment that delivers either electricity or drugs to nerves in order to change their activity.
- Sacral nerve stimulation is a means of directly stimulating the 3rd sacral nerve to alter/improve bladder and bowel function and modulate pelvic pain.
- Over the past 20 years, S3 neuromodulation has become well established as a preferred option for treatment of various disorders of the lower urogenital tract and bowel.[1-3]
- Neuromodulation includes modulation of peripheral nerve function by all means (electrical stimulation and magnetic stimulation), and also includes stimulation at any point of the nerve pathway—skin dermatomes, posterior tibial nerve and S3 neuromodulation.
- This chapter will be confined to S3 neuromodulation but the neurophysiology mechanism of action is common to all forms.

Indications

- Refractory urgency, urge incontinence
- Voiding difficulty
- Pelvic pain, vulval pain syndromes
- Fecal incontinence
- Constipation.

Anatomy and Neurophysiology

The voluntary control of micturition and defecation requires coordination of complex nerve pathways and also coordination between autonomic (parasympathetic and sympathetic) nerves and somatic nerves via the pelvic, hypogastric, and 3rd sacral nerves and the S2,3,4 sacral segments and the T11-L2 segments of the spinal cord.

Coordination is also mediated by the spinal pathways to and from those spinal segments to the midbrain and gray matter.

Sensory impulses from the bladder, rectum, vulva and pelvic floor travel as myelinated Aδ fibers and unmyelinated C fibers to the S2-4 and T11-L2 spinal cord segments. 'Normal' sensation is carried by Aδ fibers while the 'silent' C fibers are activated by noxious stimuli.

There is a dense plexus of sensory nerves in the trigonal area in the suburothelium with projections into the urothelium and probably into the detrusor muscle.

Work carried out by Professor James Gillespie confirmed that there is intrinsic bladder contractility observed in the isolated bladder possibly mediated by some of these suburothelial nerves. This activity is in the form of nonexpulsive waveform contractions throughout the bladder when the isolated bladder is placed in a physiological solution.

Myofibroblasts in the suburothelial layer may well act as stretch receptors.

It is probable that non-neuronal cells in the urothelium release transmitters such as adenosine triphosphate (ATP), acetylcholine (ACh) and NO, which can regulate the activity of adjacent nerves. There is still much work to be carried out to further elucidate the integration of these transmitters with the function of the LUGT.

Motor function of the bladder is mediated by excitatory parasympathetic outflow largely from S3 while the sympathetic outflow from T11-12 via the pudendal nerve will cause inhibition of β3 receptors in the bladder and excitation of α-adrenergic receptors in the urethra stimulating sphincter function and aiding the continence mechanism.

Neuromodulation appears to modulate these complex pathways by sensory inhibition in the spinal cord and also by modulating the ascending pathways.

There may be other modes of action not yet defined.

History of Neuromodulation

Initial attempts in the 1950s with neuromodulation and spinal cord stimulation were largely unsuccessful.

In 1981—first human implant of an S3 stimulating device was carried out with success by Tanagho and Schmidt. This was followed quickly by a successful large multicenter trial from 1985 to 1992.

Since that time there have been rapid improvements in electrodes, electrode fixation, pulse generators and techniques together with widespread acceptance and use. There have been increasing indications for the use of S3 neuromodulation.

How does Neuromodulation Work?

As described before the control of micturition and fecal and urinary continence involves complex neural networks. Subtle neuronal lesions, whether familial or acquired may result in dysfunction.

Sacral nerve stimulation (SNS) of the afferent a-delta myelinated fibers inhibits unstable neural reflex behavior and also enhances sphincter and pelvic floor activity.

The precise mechanism of action however still remains unclear.

Previous studies have shown that chronic noxious stimulation of the bladder lining—essentially what occurs in patients with IC—can cause cells in the spinal cord to overproduce an enzyme called nitric oxide synthase (NOS).

It was found that in rats with problems mimicking IC that sacral neuromodulation in an animal model reduces spinal cord expression of NOS in interstitial cystitis.

This is important because for the first time, it provides an understanding of how neuromodulation may work.

With the aid of a long fiberoptic pressure transduce with over 100 pressure sensors along its length, Phil Dinning[2] studied the activity of the large bowel and discovered reflection of peristaltic waves at the rectosigmoid junction.

Neuromodulation appeared to modulate this reflection to normalize bowel function.

Technique of S3 Neuromodulation

The technique for SNS has changed considerably over the past 17 to 18 years.

Essentially there are two stages:

1. Test phase
2. Implantation of pulse generator.

Test Phase

Peripheral Nerve Evaluation

- Initially the test was called peripheral nerve evaluation (PNE)
- A temporary single electrode is inserted via the needle electrode through the 3rd sacral foramen to stimulate 3rd sacral nerve.
- The patient is positioned prone on operating table with hips and lower legs supported and allowing toe movement to be unencumbered and readily observed.
- Buttocks taped apart and landmarks identified with a marking **(Figures 20.1 and 20.2)**.

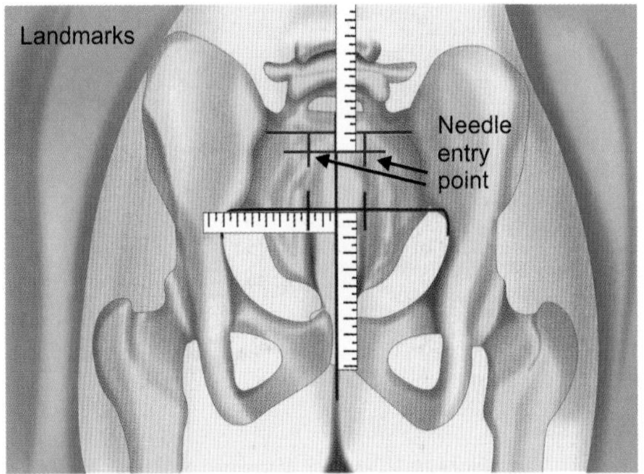

Figure 20.1: Landmarks identification with a marking

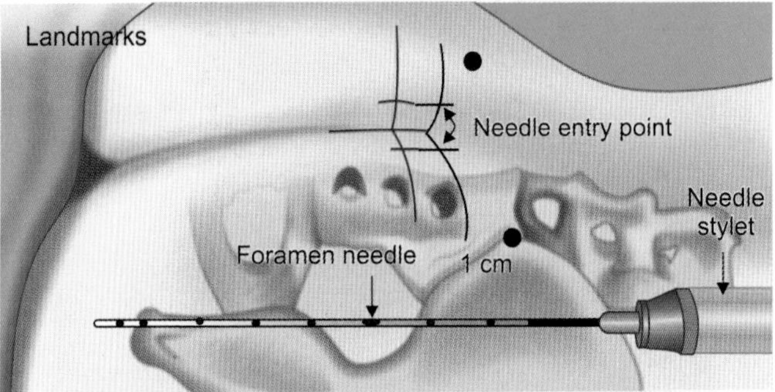

Figure 20.2: Landmarks and foramen needle

- The landmark generally 0 to 1 cm below posterior-superior ischial spine and 1 cm lateral to the midline. There are however several different approaches to obtaining this landmark.
- The foramen needle electrode inserted and checked with the image intensifier **(Figure 20.3)**.
- The needle is stimulated to check the response **(Figure 20.4)**.
- This is usually carried out under local with neurolept anesthesia but may be performed as an office procedure.
- More recently, the use of fluoroscopic imaging to assist needle and lead positioning has become imperative **(Figures 20.5A and B)**.
- There have also been improvements in the PNE lead but still migration of the lead remains very common.

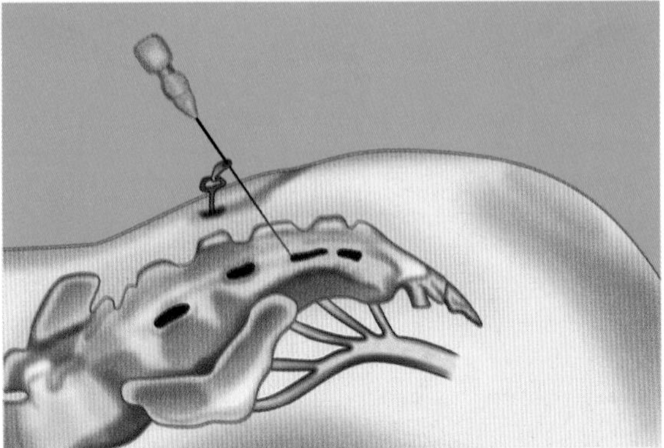

Figure 20.3: Insertion of foramen needle

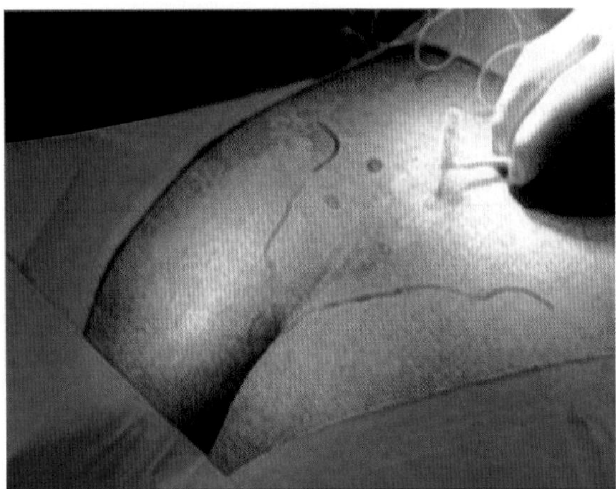

Figure 20.4: Test stimulation with the needle

- Peripheral nerve evaluation still performed in some centers but this has now largely been superseded by the staged procedure.
- After a successful test phase the PNE lead is removed and a new permanent lead is inserted, again with I/I assistance and either under GA or with local neurolept anesthetic.
- Thereafter the procedure is the same for both the PNE and the more recent 'staged' insertion

More recently, the 'tined lead' has been **(Figure 20.6)** introduced:

- This lead has fine projections which when loaded, help prevent outward migration of the lead.

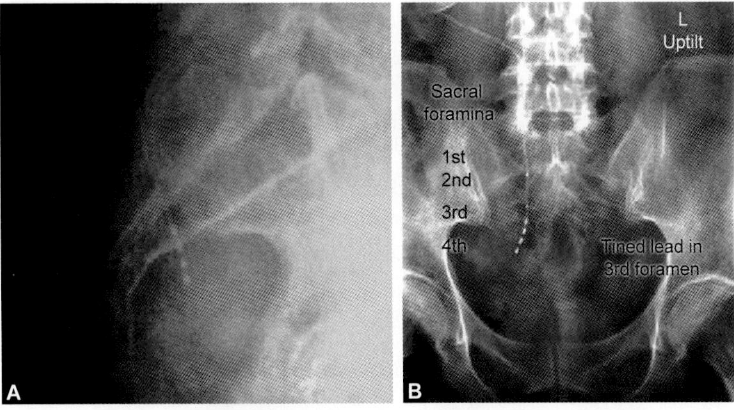

Figures 20.5A and B: X-rays of lead *in situ*

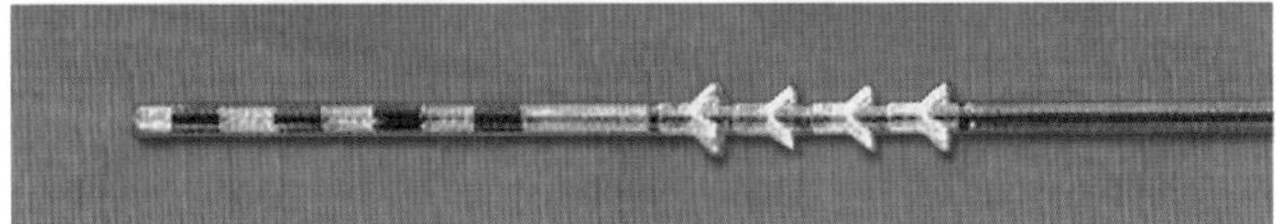

Figure 20.6: Tined lead with fine projections

- Further modifications are expected in the near future to prevent inward migration.

This is development enabled the use of the permanent tined lead in the test phase and is termed the 'staged procedure' **(Table 20.1)**.

Staged Procedure

This may be carried out with local and neurolept anesthesia although the many clinicians prefer GA. It is essential that the patient is not paralyzed as this will prevent the observation of reflex activity.

- The patient is positioned as for the PNE and the foramen needle electrode placed also in the same manner with the guidewire inserted when the electrode has been positioned correctly.
- A small skin incision (1 cm) is then made at site entrance of the electrode and the foramen needle is removed. A cannula is the inserted over the guidewire **(Figure 20.7)** and when positioned correctly the guidewire and stilette are removed. This allows insertion of the lead **(Figure 20.8)** through the cannula—again with stimulation and I/I to confirm correct placement **(Figure 20.9)**.

Table 20.1: Advantages and disadvantages of peripheral nerve evaluation (PNE)

Advantages of PNE	*Disadvantages of PNE*
Done under local with neurolept	Lead migration is extremely common
No incisions required	Lead may move as soon as the patient is moved from operating table
Minimal patient discomfort	Frequent failure of the test phase
Minimal risk of infection	Need to insert new lead for part 2 of the surgery

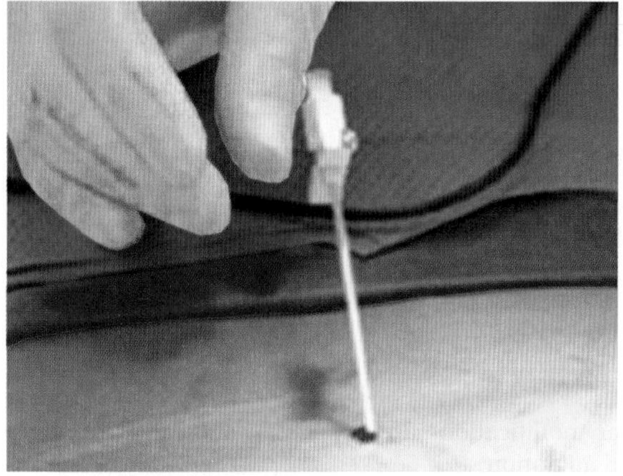

Figure 20.7: Insertion of trocar and cannula

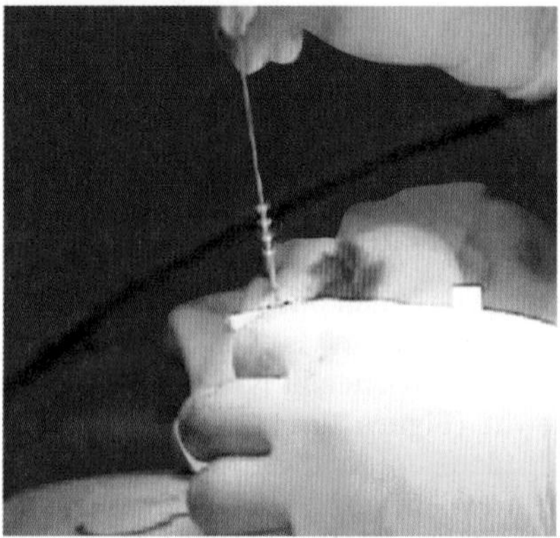

Figure 20.8: Insertion of the lead

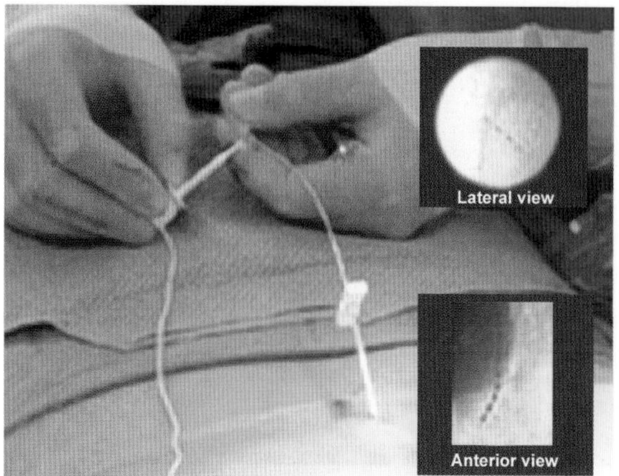

Figure 20.9: Stimulation of the lead

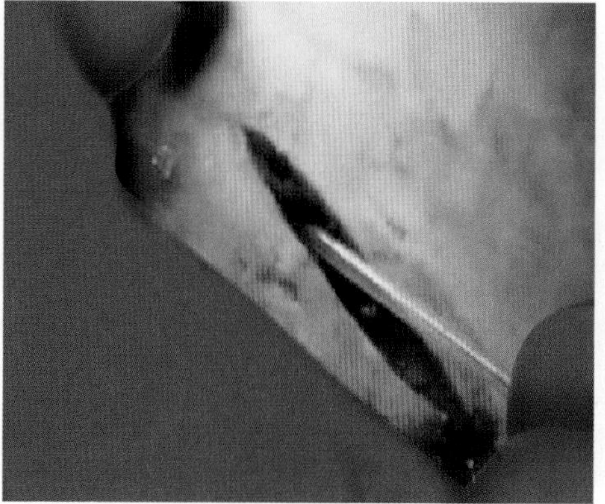

Figure 20.10: Tunneling cannula

- A right or left flank incision made and the lead tunneled to that incision **(Figure 20.10)**.
- The lead is connected to the external lead which is then tunneled to the opposite flank or further laterally on the same side and externalized ready for connection to the external pulse generator.

Second Stage

- The flank incision opened and external lead disconnected.
- A 'Pouch' for the pulse generator created and the pulse generator inserted and sutured to fascia **(Figures 20.11 and 20.12)**.

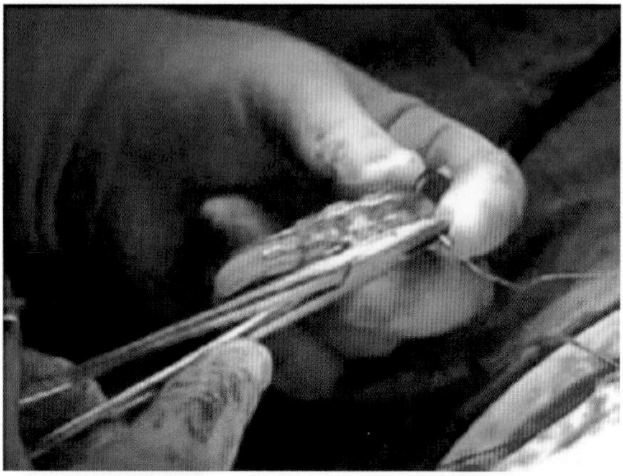

Figure 20.11: Preparing to insert pulse generator

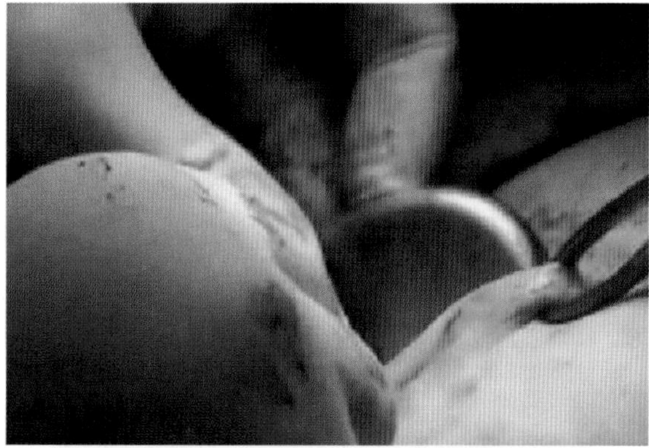

Figure 20.12: Insertion of pulse generator

The second stage may also be carried out under local and neurolept anesthesia although many including the author prefer GA. At an appropriate time after surgery, the pulse generator is programmed and when satisfactory, the patient discharged.

Should these procedures, including PNE and test stage be carried out as day case procedures?

It is important to consider that the patients having SNS have failed for some reason—previous conservative management and have very complex problems. For many of these patients, SNS is there last hope of gaining some semblance of bladder (and/or bowel) control.

Also important is that the lead is likely to migrate a little during the first 24 to 48 hours following insertion. If the lead moves and the patient has been sent home, an adequate test phase may not be obtained.

For these reasons alone the author suggests that the test phases should not be day case procedures.

Patient Selection

Patients considered for sacral neuromodulation fall into several groups:

- Refractory urgency, urge incontinence
- Voiding difficulty
- Pelvic pain, vulval pain syndromes
- Fecal incontinence
- Constipation.

Original studies excluded patients with neurogenic causes of urgency and urge incontinence of urine but experience with S3 neuromodulation in patients with neurogenic problems has increased and the response is often very satisfactory. Van Kerrebroeck has stated that while the indication for SNS in refractory idiopathic detrusor overactivity is well documented. Other authors have confirmed this[4] indication for use in the neurogenic situation is even more compelling.

Results (Figures 20.13 to 20.17)

- In most centers, the success of S3 neuromodulation for refractory lower urinary tract and bowel disorders has proven to be associated with a 70 percent success rate. This success rate is related to

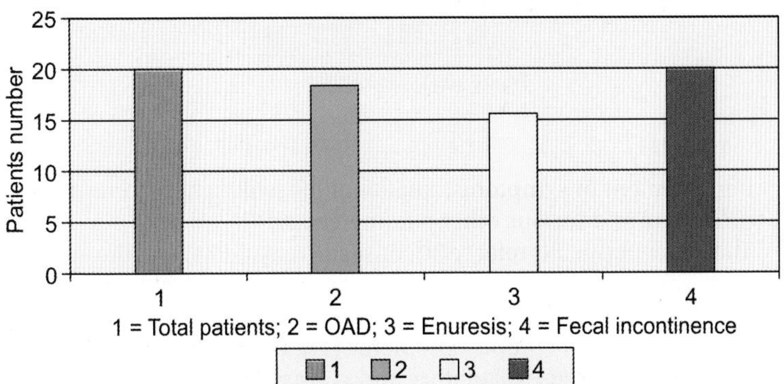

Figure 20.13: Patients number—diagnosis/problem

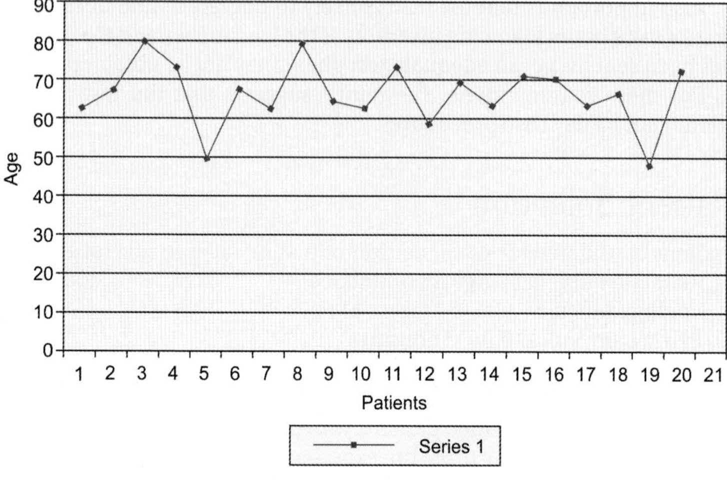

Figure 20.14: Patients age

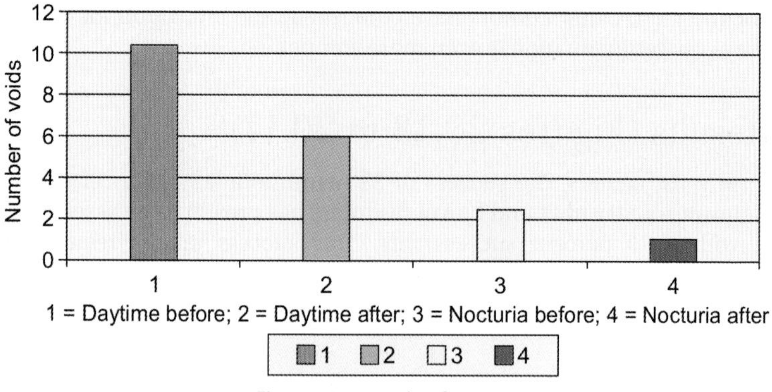

Figure 20.15: Voiding frequency

improvement in symptoms, quality of life, willingness to repeat the procedure and various other parameters.

- The following results refer to 20 consecutive patients from the author's unit—19 of whom had both refractory urinary and fecal incontinence and 2 had fecal urgency/incontinence. They represent a group of patients with very complex problems **(Figure 20.16)**.
- The results are self-explanatory and consistent with the results from most units.

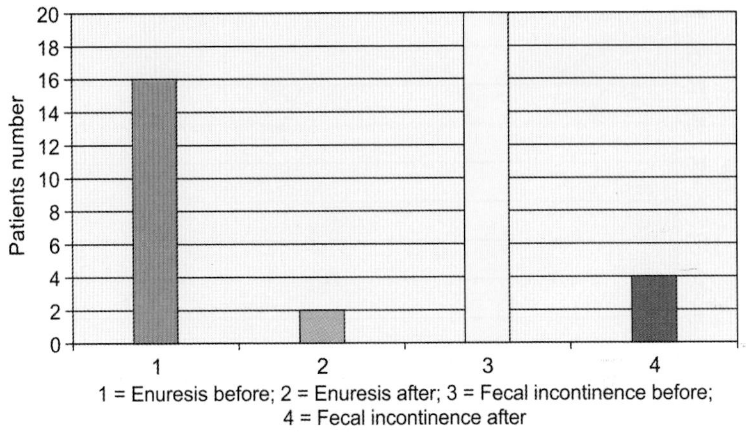

Figure 20.16: Enuresis and fecal incontinence

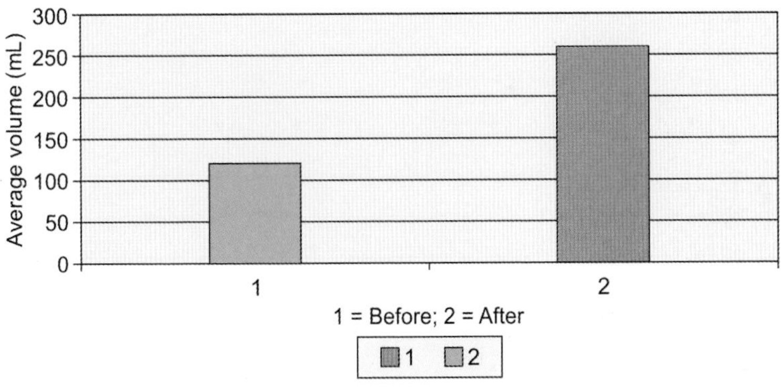

Figure 20.17: Voided volume

- These results are 2 years postoperative and long-term results (5 years) reveal very little reduction in success.

Patient Satisfaction (Figures 20.18 and 20.19)

Eighty-five percent of patients were satisfied with the procedure and outcome. There are some unexpected positive outcomes with sacral neuromodulation including improvement in global pelvic function symptoms in women.[5]

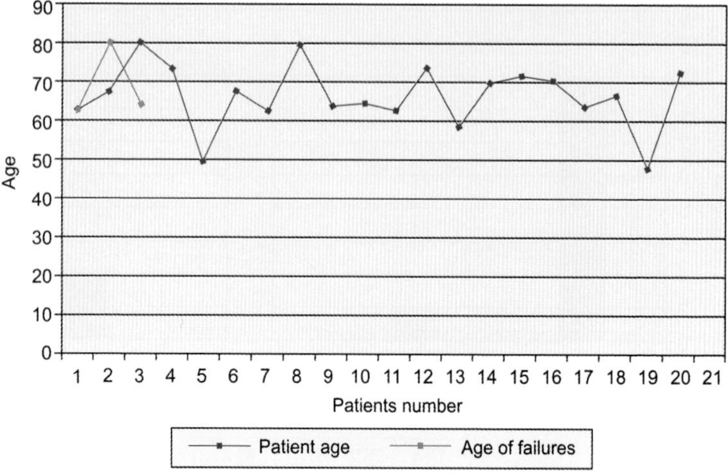

Figure 20.18: Patient age and age of failures (urine)

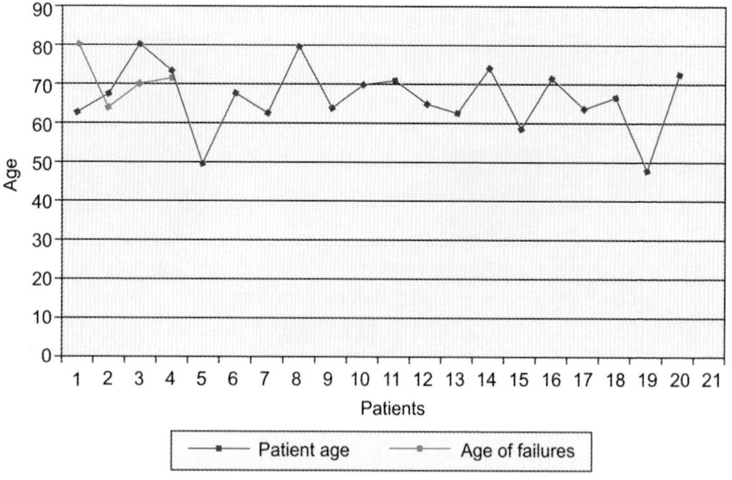

Figure 20.19: Patient age and age of failures

Cost-effectiveness

Several studies have confirmed the cost-effectiveness of S3 neuromodulation.

Complications (Figures 20.20 to 20.22)

The author has been actively utilizing S3 neuromodulation for over 18 years and has had no serious or life-threatening complications. There are however a considerable number of minor complications. These include:

- *Lead*:
  - *Lead migration—23 percent*: The lead may migrate in or out and further development is being undertaken to minimize this.

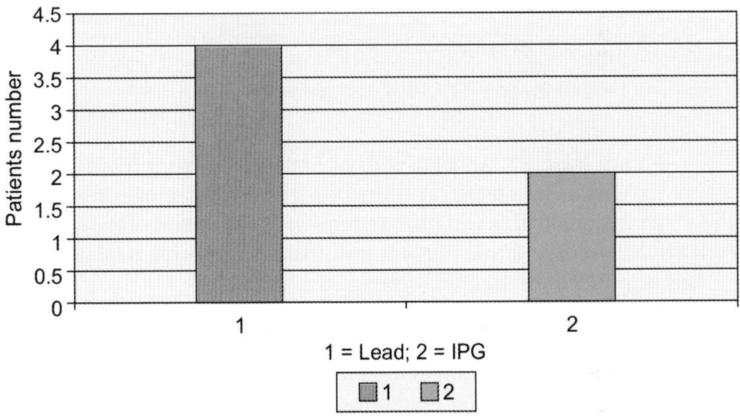

Figure 20.20: Reinsertion of lead and IPG

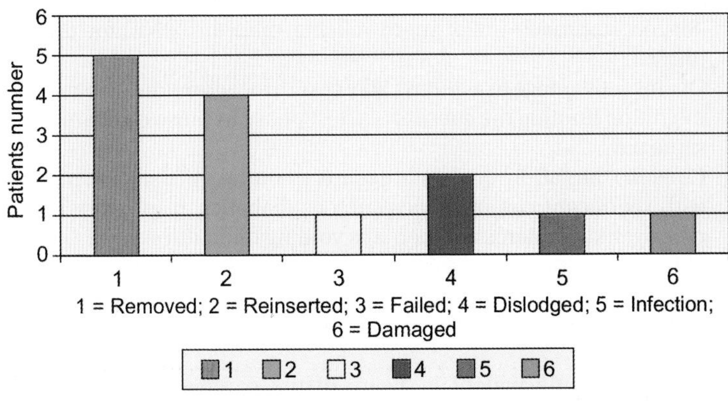

Figure 20.21: Removed/reinserted test lead—reason

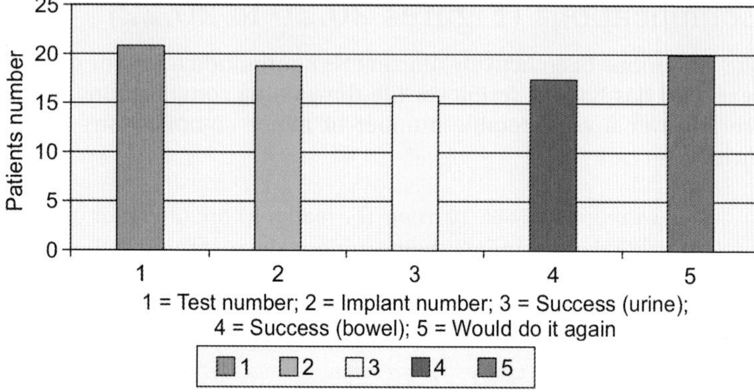

Figure 20.22: Patients number, success, and would do it again

- *Faulty lead*: Six percent with either lead fracture (complete or partial) or an electrical short between two or more electrodes. Occasionally this will require removal/reinsertion of the lead.[6]
- *Wound infection*: Three percent and usually requiring explantation. This is more common in diabetics.
- *Pulse generator*:
  - Pain at the site of the pulse generator—5 percent and occasionally requires repositioning of the pulse generator.
  - Exposure of the pulse generator—usually associated with wound infection/foreign body reaction but occasionally from trauma.

Tips and Tricks

- 'Staged' approach much more reliable than the 'PNE' for the test phase.[7]
- Distinct advantage in avoiding 'day case' procedures due to early lead migration limiting the success of a test phase in those discharged the same day.
- Consider an 'all in one' approach (i.e. no test phase) for patients with significant comorbidities such as diabetics, respiratory issues, neurogenic problems and perhaps voiding difficulties.
  This will minimize risks such as infections and anesthetic issues.
- Remember all of the patients have problems that have not responded to other treatments so, it is very important to maximize the chance of success.
- Ensure that the patient is aware of the complex nature of their problem(s) and that they have a realistic expectation of approximately 70 percent chance of significant improvement in their symptoms.

- Ensure that they are aware of possible complications such as failure, lead migration, lead fracture, pain at IPG site, and occasional need to remove and reinsert the lead.
- In refractory cases where the improvement is not adequate, consider adding medication to the treatment regime and also consider bilateral stimulation.[8]
- Use prophylactic antibiotics and continue postoperatively in diabetics or patients with debilitating disease states.
- S3 neuromodulation is safe and effective in the elderly.[9]

Who Should do this Procedure?

S3 neuromodulation is reserved at this stage for patients with very complex problems. It is appropriate that those performing this procedure are either subspecialists or working in tertiary units.

There are considerable differences in the availability of such services between health care regions and between different countries. It is therefore, difficult to be more specific but the above principles should be entertained.

Future

- The field of neuromodulation is constantly expanding.
- Posterior tibial nerve stimulation, pudendal nerve stimulation and tens are examples of other forms of neuromodulation.
- Neuromodulation of bladder activity by stimulation of feline pudendal nerve using a transdermal amplitude modulated signal (TAMS) is a recent development.
- This application is still in developmental phase.
- Further improvements in the S3 lead are likely in the near future and ability to program 'On-line' is desperately needed.
- The availability of pulse generators (IPGs) that are not receptive to the MRI frequencies will enable the procedure to be more readily utilized in patients who are likely to require MRI scanning.
- There is an urgent need to upgrade the electronics to enable 'on-line' programming of the pulse generator and a 'bluetooth' or similar connection from the pulse generator to a computer.

Summary

S3 neuromodulation has been carried out for over two decades and is a safe reliable and cost-effective means of improving the symptoms in a large group of patients who have failed to respond to other treatment modalities. S3 neuromodulation is life-changing in those successful patients.

References

1. Clare J Fowler, Derek Griffiths, William C de Groat. The neural control of micturition. The publisher's final edited version of this article is available at Nat Rev Neurosci.
2. The autonomous bladder: a view of the origin of bladder overactivity and sensory urge. BJU International Volume 93, 2004.
3. Patton V, Wiklendt L, Arkwright JW, Lubowski DZ, Dinning PG. The effect of sacral nerve stimulation on distal colonic motility in patients with faecal incontinence. Br J Surg. 2013 Mar 27. doi: 10.1002/bjs.9114.
4. Chaabane W, Guillotreau J, Castel- Lacanal E, Abu-Anz S, De Boissezon X, Malavaud B, Marque P, Sarramon JP, Rischmann P, Game X. Sacral neuromodulation for treating neurogenic bladder dysfunction: clinical and urodynamic study. Service d'Urologie, Andrologie et Transplantation Rénale, Toulouse, France. Neurourol Urodyn. 2011;30(4):547-50. doi: 10.1002/nau.21009.
5. Jadav AM, Wadhawan H, Jones GL, Wheldon LW, Radley SC, Brown SR. Does sacral nerve stimulation improve global pelvic function in women? Colorectal Dis. 2013 Mar 2. doi: 10.1111/codi.12181.
6. Lenis AT, Gill BC, Carmel ME, Rajki M, Moore CK, Vasavada SP, Goldman HB, Rackley RR. Patterns of Hardware Related Electrode Failures in Sacral Nerve Stimulation. J Urol. 2013 Jan 9. pii: S0022-5347(13)00038-4. doi: 10.1016/j.juro.2013.01.013.
7. Chad Baxter, Ja-Hong Kim. Contrasting the Percutaneous Nerve Evaluation Versus Staged Implantation in Sacral Neuromodulation. Curr Urol Rep. 2010;11(5):310-4. Published online 2010 June 10. doi: 10.1007/s11934-010-0128-2.
8. Marcelissen TA, Leong RK, Serroyen J, van Kerrebroeck PE, De Wachter SG. The use of bilateral sacral nerve stimulation in patients with loss of unilateral treatment efficacy. Department of Urology, Maastricht University Medical Centre, Maastricht, The Netherlands.
9. Pettit PD, Chen A. Implantable neuromodulation for urinary urge incontinence and fecal incontinence: a urogynecology perspective. Department of Gynecologic Surgery, Mayo Clinic Florida, Jacksonville, FL 32224, USA. *paul.pettit@mayo.edu.*

Appendix

Policy

Some units demand a 'Policy' for procedures. The following is a Policy that is often used:

Urinary incontinence and nonobstructive retention:

A. A trial period of sacral nerve neuromodulation with either percutaneous nerve stimulation or a temporarily implanted lead may be considered medically necessary in patients who meet all of the following criteria:
   1. There is a diagnosis of at least one of the following:
      a. Urge incontinence
      b. Urgency-frequency
      c. Nonobstructive urinary retention
   2. There is documented failure or intolerance to at least two conventional therapies (e.g. behavioral training such as bladder training, prompted voiding, or pelvic muscle exercise training, pharmacologic treatment for at least a sufficient duration to fully assess its efficacy, and/or surgical corrective therapy).

B. Permanent implantation of a sacral nerve neuromodulation device may be considered medically necessary in patients who meet all of the following criteria:
   1. All of the criteria in A (1–2) above are met.
   2. A trial stimulation period demonstrates at least 50 percent improvement in symptoms over a period of at least 2 weeks.

Sacral nerve neuromodulation may be considered medically necessary for the treatment of fecal incontinence when all of the following criteria are met:

1. Chronic fecal incontinence of greater than 2 incontinent episodes on average per week with duration greater than 6 months or for more than 12 months after vaginal childbirth.
2. Documented failure or intolerance to conventional therapy [e.g. dietary modification, the addition of bulking and pharmacologic treatment for at least a sufficient duration to fully assess its efficacy, and/or surgical corrective therapy performed more than 12 months (or 24 months in case of cancer) previously].
3. The patient is an appropriate surgical candidate.
4. A successful percutaneous test stimulation, defined as at least 50 percent improvement in symptoms, was performed (This should not necessarily be a strict criteria as any improvement in the test phase may be worthwhile).

Artificial Urinary Sphincter in the Management of Severe Intrinsic Sphincter Deficiency Incontinence in Women

Vincent Tse, Li-Tsa Koh

Introduction

Currently, the midurethral synthetic sling (MUS) is the gold standard in the management of female urodynamic stress urinary incontinence (USUI). It has a high success rate in primary as well as recurrent USUI with long-term follow-up to 10 years or more.[1-3] Although earlier studies on the MUS had shown the retropubic approach to be equivalent to the transobturator route with respect to efficacy, more recent data had revealed that in patients with predominately intrinsic sphincter deficiency (ISD), the retropubic approach is more effective.[4] In patients who failed a previous MUS, many authors have shown that after careful urodynamic evaluation, a repeat retropubic MUS or a fascial pubovaginal sling would be useful.[5] However, if this second sling fails, there is little data to show that further repeat slings would be of value in rendering continence. Therefore, in clinical practice, there remains a small patient cohort who will fail currently available sling procedures due to severe ISD and will require more invasive salvage procedures. One such option is the artificial urinary sphincter which has been shown, over many years, to improve continence and quality of life in this difficult patient group.[6] This chapter will focus on the use of this device.

Nature and Mechanism of Action

The most widely used artificial urinary sphincter is designed and manufactured by American Medical Systems, (Minnetonka, USA). Its prototype was developed in the late 1970s, and had undergone multiple refinements to its present form, model the AMS-800™. It is a solid silicone elastomer device which includes a fluid filled cuff, a control pump and a pressure-regulating balloon. These three components are connected to each other with kink-resistant tubing (**Figure 21.1**).

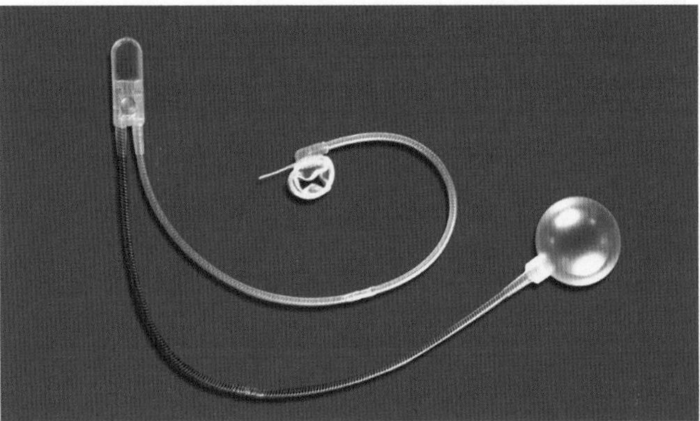

Figure 21.1: The AMS 800 artificial urinary sphincter showing the circular fluid-filled cuff, spherical fluid reservoir, and the control pump (with permission to use from American Medical Systems, Minnetonka, USA)

The cuff is placed around the urethra (or bladder neck if clinically indicated) and it compresses on and occludes the urethra when it is filled with fluid, mimicking the action of the urinary sphincter. The compression of the urethra enables the patient to remain continent. When there is a desire to void, the patient squeezes the control pump placed inside the labial fat to transfer fluid from the cuff to the pressure-regulating balloon which is usually implanted in the suprapubic region behind the rectus abdominis muscle. This allows the cuff to empty, removing the compression on the urethra. Urine will then pass freely down the urethra. After approximately three minutes, fluid automatically shifts from the balloon to the cuff. When the cuff is filled, it compresses on the urethra to once again provide continence.

Clinical Indications

The artificial urinary sphincter (AUS) is not a first-line procedure for stress incontinence. Its place in the management of stress incontinence comes as a salvage procedure, often after multiple sling failures in the setting of a fixed nonmobile urethra on fluoroscopic or ultrasound guided urodynamics, together with a very low maximum urethral closure pressure (MUCP) often less than 10 cm H_2O, or a very low abdominal leak point pressure (ALPP) often less than 30 cm H_2O.[7] The patient often reports continuous profuse leakage during the daytime with little or no rise in intra-abdominal pressure, as well as during sleep. The patient should have a reasonable degree of manual dexterity and a good working knowledge of the device prior to surgery. The informed consent should include a discussion involving the success and failure rates, revision rate, risk of device malfunction, erosion, and infection.

Contraindications and Caveats

Caution has to be exercised when contemplating implantation of the artificial urinary sphincter if one of the following conditions exist:

- Pre-existing physical or mental co-morbidities that may preclude the patient to surgery and anesthesia
- Refractory detrusor overactivity or poor bladder compliance as the implantation may exacerbate the problem and put the upper renal tract at risk
- Urinary incontinence due to or complicated by an irreversibly obstructed lower urinary tract
- Untreated bladder outlet obstruction such as urethral stricture or bladder neck contracture
- Previous pelvic radiotherapy is generally considered a relative contraindication due to the statistically higher rates of postoperative infections and erosions
- Poor manual dexterity that may affect the ability of the patient to operate the pump
- Patients with poor motivation to operate the AUS
- Physical limitations of the patient such as arthritis and morbid obesity that may affect the ability of the patient to access the implanted pump
- Allergy or sensitivity to the Rifampin, Minocycline or other tetracyclines.[8,9]

Measures should be taken to treat any existing infection to reduce the risk of infection of the implanted device. A poorly compliant or small fibrotic bladder may require some intervention before the implantation as well. Another relative contraindication would be a personal history of bladder malignancies or urolithiasis where frequent urethral instrumentations may be necessary.

Operative Technique

The procedure should be undertaken by a urologist with expertise in the field of prosthetics as well as in the management of failed slings. A good understanding of surgical anatomy of the pelvis is crucial as these patients often have complicated and distorted pelvic anatomy due to multiple past transvaginal, retropubic, as well as periurethral procedures. As it involves implantation of a prosthesis, it is imperative that surgical asepsis is enforced. Preoperative urine culture should be sterile. Intravenous antibiotics covering skin gram positive cocci and enterobacteriaceae should be used, such as vancomycin and an aminoglycoside, respectively. Traffic should be minimized in an out of the operating room during the case to minimize aerosolized bacteria settling on the prosthesis or surgical wounds. Skin at the operative site should be scrubbed for between 5 and 10 minutes with povidone-iodine, then air-dry, prior to skin-prepping and incision. In the female, the most commonly used approach is a lower midline abdominal or Pfennenstiel incision. This is to allow cuff placement around the bladder neck, with the operating pump sited in the subcutaneous fat pad in the labium major. This fat pad can be accessed by blunt dissection in the subcutaneous fat just superficial and medial to the superficial inguinal ring. The pressure-regulating reservoir can be placed in the retropubic space adjacent to the bladder (**Figure 21.2**). Meticulous attention is necessary during dissection to achieve a plane between the bladder neck and anterior vaginal wall, to avoid perforation of the bladder and vagina. In those patients who had had a previous sling procedure, the location of this plane may be aided by following the path of the previously placed sling towards the bladder neck. Once the plane is achieved, the cuff sizer is placed around the bladder neck (**Figure 21.3**) to measure the most appropriate cuff size to effect a mucosal seal without causing excessive constriction around the bladder neck which may increase the risk of

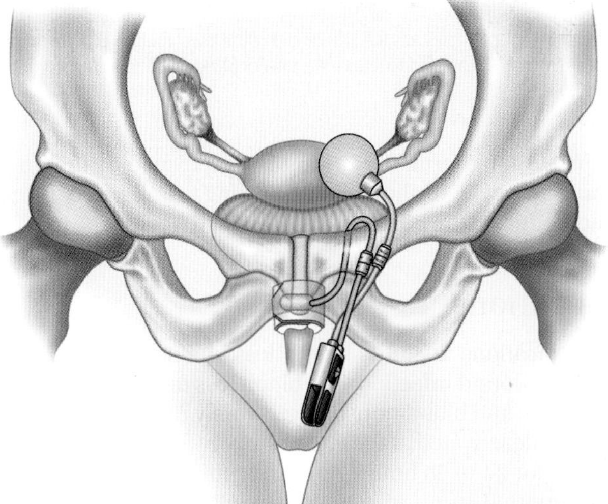

Figure 21.2: Pictorial representation of how the AMS 800 sphincter system would look like after implantation in the female. The cuff is around the bladder neck, the spherical reservoir in the retropubic space adjacent to the bladder, and the control pump in the labium major. All three components are connected by kink-resistant tubing in a closed system (with permission to use from American Medical Systems, Minnetonka, USA)

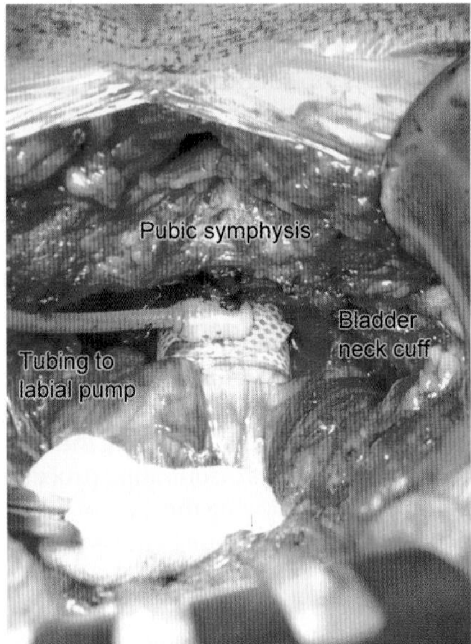

Figure 21.3: Intraoperative photograph showing the sphincter cuff around the bladder neck in a 44-year-old female with severe intrinsic sphincter deficiency after repair of a urethro-vaginal fistula. She had failed a midurethral synthetic sling as well as an autologous rectus fascia pubovaginal sling. The top of the photograph represents the inferior end of the lower midline abdominal incision. The sponge in the foreground was used to retract the anterior bladder wall to aid in demonstrating the bladder neck cuff

erosion in the long-term. The pump is deactivated at the end of the operation for 6 weeks, to allow wound healing to take place. The surgeon reactivates it during the postoperative visit at 6 weeks.

Complications

Early complications include blood loss, hematoma, pain, urinary retention and wound infection. The blood loss during surgery is usually less than 50 mL and blood transfusion is rarely required.[10]

The cuff is deactivated at the end of surgery and the patient is usually catheterized for 24 to 48 hours. Acute retention following implantation has been reported in up to 4 to 20 percent of patients. If the patient develops urinary retention, one should check that the cuff has been deactivated. An image guided suprapubic approach to catheterize the patient is preferred if the patient is unable to void after 48 hours as an indwelling urethral catheter would increase the incidence of urethral erosion. A urodynamic study should be performed in the case of persistent urinary retention after a few weeks. A repeat surgery with a resized cuff may be necessary if the retention was shown to be due to an undersized cuff.

Postoperative implant infection rates have been reported to be about 5 percent while urinary infection rates have been reported in up to 23 percent of patients. Higher implant infection rates of up to 10 percent have been reported in cases with prior irradiation and previous failed surgical procedures. *Staphylococcus aureus* and *Staphylococcus epidermidis* are the usual organisms responsible for infections and prophylactic antibiotics with adequate coverage should be given during surgery. The development of the InhibiZone® surface treatment should lead to lower reported infection rates in the coming years.[11]

Late complications include the development of overactive bladder, urethral erosion, vaginal erosion, labia major erosion, bladder erosion, urethral stricture, urethral atrophy and mechanical failure of the device. The development of *de novo* overactive bladder has been reported in up to 10 percent of patients which can be treated with anticholinergic agents or intradetrusor injection of botulinum toxin.

Current literature reports urethral erosion rate to be about 5 to 10 percent. Urethral erosion and infection are closely related and inevitably lead to explantation of the AUS. The incidence of pressure induced ischemia and necrosis has been greatly reduced since the introduction of postoperative deactivation of the AUS by Furlow and Barrett.[12] Risk factors of erosion and explantation include age >70, a history of smoking, previous surgery and irradiation.[13]

The mean mechanical survival of the AUS has been found to be about 15 years. Significant factors affecting survival include the number of previous surgeries and if the patient had a neurological indication for the AUS. Patients with 2 or more previous surgeries and patients with neurogenic bladders were at a significantly higher risk for mechanical failure.[14]

Clinical Efficacy

The AUS can be useful in improving quality of life in the difficult patient with a devastated outlet after multiple sling failures.[15,16] Chung et al reviewed cases at their unit over a 25-year period. A total of 29 female patients received AUS following failed anti-incontinence surgeries. There was a significant reduction in pad usage (3.6 to 0.2 pads per day; $p < 0.01$). The continence rate with no pad was 70 percent and this increases to 83 percent in patients wearing one precautionary pad. Five (17%) AUS devices were explanted due to AUS erosion or infection. Thirteen AUS revisions were made and device malfunction accounted for 95 percent of the cases. Kaplan-Meier analysis showed more than 90 percent of AUS malfunction occurred less than 100 months from the time of implant. The authors concluded that the AUS is a safe, durable and effective salvage procedure in the patient with multiple sling failure in the presence of severe compromise to urethral and rhabdosphincter function.[7]

Conclusion

The artificial urinary sphincter is a salvage procedure which can be effectively used in patients with a devastated outlet who had, by and large, completely lost urethral sphincter function. It should be considered in patients who had failed two or more of the conventional sling procedures such as the MUS or the pubovaginal sling, as further sling will most likely not be beneficial to effect continence, and may make future AUS implantation potentially more difficult. It should be performed by a urologist with ample experience in the assessment and management of complicated bladder dysfunction. These patients will require life-long follow-up as there is a likelihood that revision surgery will be required in the future, for malfunction from frequent usage, or for complications such as cuff erosion or urethral atrophy. Many patients with severe sphincter deficiency and failed slings are currently managed with some form of permanent catheterization such as a suprapubic catheter. However, it is important to note that the AUS can be an option in these cases, and referrals should be made to those urologists who are proficient in its use, so that women with sling-refractory intrinsic sphincter deficiency incontinence can be salvaged to improve their quality of life, and avoid permanent catheterization.

References

1. Nilsson CG, Palva K, Aarnio R, Morcos E, Falconer C. Seventeen years follow-up of the tension-free vaginal tape procedure for female stress urinary incontinence. Int Urogynecol J. 2013 Apr 6. [Epub ahead of print]
2. Chung E, Tse V, Chan L. Midurethral synthetic slings in the treatment of urodynamic female stress urinary incontinence without concomitant pelvic prolapse repair: 4-year health-related quality of life outcomes. BJU Int. 2010;105(4):514-7.
3. Svenningsen R, Staff AC, Schiøtz HA, Western K, Kulseng-Hanssen S. Long-term follow-up of the retropubic tension-free vaginal tape procedure. Int Urogynecol J. 2013 Feb 16. [Epub ahead of print]
4. Schierlitz L, Dwyer PL, Rosamilia A, Murray C, Thomas E, De Souza A, Hiscock R. Three-year follow-up of tension-free vaginal tape compared

with transobturator tape in women with stress urinary incontinence and intrinsic sphincter deficiency. Obstet Gynecol. 2012;119 (2 Pt 1):321-7.

5. Welk BK, Herschorn S. The autologous fascia pubovaginal sling for complicated female stress incontinence. Can Urol Assoc J. 2012;6(1):36-40.
6. Eric Chung, Ross A. Cartmill. Twenty-five years experience in the outcome of artificial urinary sphincter in the treatment of female urinary incontinence. BJU Int. 2010;106:1664-7.
7. Rea D, Lavelle J, Carson C III. Chapter 14, Artificial Urethral Sphincters. In: The Bionic Human, Edited by Johnson and Virgo, Humana Press; 2006.pp.313-21.
8. Chartier-Kastler E, Van Kerrebroeck P, et al. Artificial urinary sphincter (AMS800) implantation for women with instrinsic sphincter deficiency: a technique for insiders? BJU Int. 2011;107(10):1618-26.
9. Wessells H, Peterson A. Artificial Urinary Sphincter and Male Perineal Sling. Chapter 79. Campbell-Walsh Urology, 10th edn. In: W Scott McDougal, Alan J Wein, Louis R Kavoussi, Andrew C Novick, Alan W Partin, Craig A Peters, Parvati Ramchandani (Eds), Elsevier saunders, 2011.
10. Thomas K, Venn SN, Mundy AR. Outcome of the artificial urinary sphincter in female patients. J Urol. 2002;167:1720-2.
11. Pierre Costa, Gregoire Poinas, et al. Long-term results of artificial urinary sphincter for women with type III stress urinary incontinence. Eur Urology. 2013;64(4):753-8.
12. Furlow WL, Barrett DM. The artificial urinary sphincter: experience with the AS 800 pump-control assembly for single-stage primary deactivation and activation—a preliminary report. Mayo Clin Proc. 1985;60:255-8.
13. Bertrand Vayleux, Jerome Rigaud, et al. Female urinary incontinence and artificial urinary sphincter: Study of efficacy and risk factors for failure and complications. Eur Urology. 2011;59(6):1048-53.
14. Chung E, Navaratnam A, Cartmill RA. Can artificial urinary sphincter be an effective salvage option in women following failed anti-incontinence surgery? Int Urogynecol J. 2011;22(3):363-6.
15. Phé V, Rouprêt M, Mozer P, Chartier-Kastler E. Trends in the landscape of artificial urinary sphincter implantation in men and women in France over the past decade. Eur Urol. 2013;63(2):407-8.
16. Revaux A, Rouprêt M, Seringe E, Misraï V, Cour F, Chartier-Kastler E. Is the implantation of an artificial urinary sphincter with a large cuff in women with severe urinary incontinence associated with worse perioperative complications and functional outcomes than usual? Int Urogynecol J. 2011;22(10):1319-24.

Index

Page numbers followed by *f* refer to figure and *t* refer to table

D

E

F

G

H

I

K

L

M

N

O

P

U

V

W